William Vayda is one of Austral
He specialises in environmental and nutritional medicine, particularly in the treatment of Chronic Fatigue Syndrome, post-viral syndromes, psychiatric disorders related to nutritional problems (orthomolecular psychiatry) and disorders of immunity, especially allergies, candida, arthritis, asthma, and related conditions.

A graduate osteopath, Dr Vayda first became interested in the role of nutrition in psychiatry. He obtained postgraduate diplomas in nutrition-naturopathy, acupuncture and clinical hypnotherapy, and was appointed senior lecturer in physiology, differential diagnosis and clinical nutrition at the Sydney College of Chiropractic and Osteopathy in 1973. The following year he founded the Australian Institute for Orthomolecular Research in Sydney. For many years he specialised in the nutritional treatment of psychiatric problems and later became interested in the role of allergies in human illness, the effects of latent viral diseases and the impacts of chemicals on human health.

He continued to lecture at universities, medical schools and various naturopathic colleges, as well as to the general public. Then, in the late 1970s, he began a program of training for medical doctors and other health professionals and ran special postgraduate courses in nutritional and environmental medicine (clinical ecology) and psychiatry, which provided the impetus for the development of a complementary approach to medicine in Australia. Working as a clinician and diagnostician with a group of medical scientists, Dr Vayda carried out extensive research into the role of latent viruses and toxic chemicals in Chronic Fatigue Syndrome and other immunological disorders.

As an adviser to a leading Australian pathology group, he helped foster the introduction of specialised tests for the assessment of viral activity, nutritional balance, chemical sensitivity and immunology. Working with Drs Mark Donohoe, Alex Taylor, Joachim Fluherer and Barry Ryan, in 1988 Dr Vayda produced the first scientific evidence of the role of chemical overloading in a group of Chronic Fatigue patients.

Dr Vayda is the President of the International College of Applied Nutrition (Australia), and a member of the Australasian Society of Osteopaths, the Complementary Medicine Association, the International Academy of Preventive Medicine, the Academy of Orthomolecular Psychiatry, the Huxley Institute for Biosocial Research and the Australian Natural Therapists Association (ANTA).

A well-known and prolific writer, Dr Vayda's weekly health column appeared in the Sydney *Sun* for many years. He was nutrition and science editor of *Nature and Health* magazine and is now contributing editor of *Wellbeing* magazine. William Vayda's 'Dear Alternative Doctor' columns and scientific articles are often published in Australian periodicals and he appears frequently on radio and television.

A pioneer of research into allergy syndromes, Dr Vayda wrote Australia's first book on the subject, *Are You Allergic to the Twentieth Century?* (1980), which was followed by *The Candida Questions and Answer Book* in 1989.

William Vayda is in private practice at the Complementary and Environmental Medicine Centre in Sydney and works as a consultant at a medical centre at Surfers Paradise, Queensland.

To Fiorella

Chronic Fatigue

The Silent Epidemic

William Vayda

With contributions from
Dr Mark Donohoe, Dr Mark Florence, Dr Peter Dobie
and Dr Michael Glasby

SIMON & SCHUSTER
AUSTRALIA

First published in Australasia in 1991 by
Simon & Schuster Australia
20 Barcoo Street, East Roseville NSW 2069
Reprinted 1992
A Paramount Communications Company
Sydney   New York   London   Toronto   Tokyo   Singapore

Text © 1991 Dr William Vayda
Illustrations © 1991 Simon & Schuster Australia

All rights reserved. No part of this publication may be reproduced, stored in a retrieval system, or transmitted, in any form or by any means, electronic, mechanical, photocopying, recording or otherwise, without the prior permission of the publisher in writing.

National Library of Australia
Cataloguing in Publication data

Vayda, William, 1930– .
Chronic fatigue.

Includes index.
ISBN 0 7318 0238 1.

1. Chronic fatigue syndrome — Popular works.
I. Title.

616.047

Designed by Kathie Baxter Smith, Design Smiths
All cartoons by Allan Stomann
Typeset in Australia by Asset Typesetting Pty Limited
Printed in Australia by the Australian Print Group

Foreword

Chronic Fatigue Syndrome (CFS) is a modern disease that is only just beginning to be accepted as a reality by conventional medical practitioners. It is a debilitating condition that is causing suffering to many thousands of Australians and preventing them from enjoying life to the full. CFS is not simply feeling a little tired for much of the time; it is an *overwhelming* tiredness that requires a major effort to drag yourself out of bed and carry out simple tasks. It saps your energy, your initiative, your sense of humour, and destroys your relationships with other people. It is not clear exactly why CFS has emerged as a new disease. Clearly, it is caused by a breakdown in the immune system, and immune deficiency diseases appear to be increasing rapidly in recent years. These conditions range from those such as allergies, where a relatively small depression of the immune system is involved, to AIDS, where immunity is highly compromised.

Various theories have been proposed to explain the modern prevalence of immune deficiency diseases; these theories include poor nutrition, pesticides, food additives, indoor air pollution, multiplication of viral infections, electromagnetic radiation, and high intake of polyunsaturated fats. It may be one or more of these factors, or some other function of modern life. Once CFS has been fully accepted as a real disease by the medical establishment, large-scale research programs can be initiated to find the cause, or causes, of the disease.

Dr William Vayda is a world expert on CFS, and has treated hundreds of patients with the condition. His extensive study and experience of CFS symptoms, and the continuous fine tuning of his treatment procedure allow him to write this authoritative and highly readable book on the subject. The text is written in a style that is readily understood by the layperson, yet contains a great deal of information for the serious student.

However, this book is much more than a treatise on CFS. It presents an holistic approach to the prevention and treatment of disease, and explains why modern, Western, clinically-based medicine so often fails to cure chronic illness. Preventive medicine has been sadly neglected in Western medical training, yet surely the true art of medicine lies in the ability to prevent, rather than treat, disease.

We are an ageing society. By the turn of the century, one person in seven will be aged over 65 years, yet these extra years are not always happy ones because many aged people suffer from a variety of debilitating chronic diseases. It is obviously better to prevent these diseases rather than treat them in an ad hoc manner as they appear. To make preventive medicine effective, there must be collaboration between medical practitioners and practitioners of complementary medicine. Both of these groups must accept that they have a duty to inform and educate the public so that everyone can accept responsibility for controlling their own health. This book is a major contribution towards achieving that goal.

T. Mark Florence, MSc., DSc., FRACI
Director, Centre for Environmental and Health Science
Formerly Chief Research Scientist, CSIRO

Foreword

Fatigue is one of the commonest symptoms heard by any health practitioner. As a clinician practising in the field of environmental medicine, I see increasing numbers of patients complaining of being 'exhausted' or of being 'tired all the time'.

The causes of fatigue are many and varied. Most people will feel somewhat tired at the end of a hard day's work, but a whole host of physical and psychological factors can combine to cause tiredness out of proportion to effort expended.

Most doctors have a few patients with a long list of symptoms, including fatigue, who defy conventional attempts at medical diagnosis. Less enlightened physicians have tended to reach for their referral pads and send such people in the direction of a psychiatrist. In recent years, more and more doctors have recognised that a large proportion of such patients do in fact have a physical basis to their illness, and we have seen the advent of the diagnosis 'Chronic Fatigue Syndrome'.

Environmental medicine, otherwise known as clinical ecology, is an orientation in medicine concerned with the role of environmental factors in illness. Increasingly, it is being demonstrated that environmental influences are important in many cases of Chronic Fatigue Syndrome.

Clinical ecologist Dr William Vayda has had extensive experience in the recognition and treatment of Chronic Fatigue Syndrome. Dr

Vayda's concepts of the nature of this disorder are reasoned and scientific, and are based on his assessment of many thousands of patients, and on his exhaustive knowledge of nutritional and environmental medicine. It is timely that with this book Dr Vayda has chosen to share with the public the benefit of his many years of clinical observation and research.

> Dr Peter Dobie, MB, BS, BMed Sci
> Environmental Medicine Centre
> Manly Waters Private Hospital
> Manly, NSW

Acknowledgements

Many people have contributed directly and indirectly to this book — too many to mention them all. Be that as it may, *Chronic Fatigue* would not have been possible without the inspiration, writing and teachings of many great scientists from whom I have learnt so much. The original inspiration was provided by those great Australians, Drs Archie Kalokerinos, Glen Dettman and Chris Reading. The writing and lecturing of, and personal contacts with, the fathers of orthomolecular (nutritional) psychiatry and medicine, Drs Abraham Hoffer and Roger Williams, over a quarter of a century taught me much of what forms the basis of anything I teach, lecture or write about. Drs Bernard Rimland, Sherry Rogers, Carl Pfeiffer, T. Randolph and William Rae taught me much over the years, but much of the original credit must go to Dr Richard Mackarness whose teachings first alerted us to the role of nutrition and allergies/intolerances as well as chemical overloading in human illness. The help, contributions and personal as well as professional friendships with Drs Treacy, Donohoe and Glasby have been invaluable, as have the continuous interactions with scientists such as Mark Florence and Greg Miller. I thank them all.

Contents

Introduction	11
OUR BODIES — OUR ENVIRONMENT	
Environmental Medicine and Total Load	17
The Immune System	19
Biochemical Individuality	34
Foods for Moods	42
Stress	45
CFS — AN OVERVIEW	
Just What is CFS?	54
The CFS Puzzle	55
Do I Have CFS?	63
VIRAL CFS	
The Viral Story	74
Epstein Barr Virus	76
Diagnosis	85
The Liver	87
CHEMICAL CFS	
Your Environment	91
Are You Tired or Toxic?	100
Neurotoxins	112
Pesticides	126
What You Can Do to Help Yourself	132
ILLNESS AND COMPLICATIONS ASSOCIATED WITH CFS	
Allergies and CFS	138
Candida and CFS	149
APICHS — Another Form of CFS	169
Depression and CFS	172
Weight Problems and CFS	181
TREATING CFS	194

DOCTORS TALK TO DOCTORS ABOUT CFS
Dr Mark Donohoe   208
Dr Michael Glasby   232

HOW TO INTERPRET VIRAL CFS READINGS   245

SOME USEFUL ADDRESSES   246
GLOSSARY   247
BIBLIOGRAPHY   251
INDEX   253

Introduction

After practising orthomolecular medicine and clinical ecology for the best part of 20 years, I found myself in a curious position. Looking back on my experience I realised that every few years a new 'disease' was discovered and became fashionable. Each of these new diseases was deemed to be the *real* cause of the problems which patients complained of. Some of you may recall the days when it was believed that hypoglycaemia was a disease in itself, and indeed was thought to be the underlying 'cause' of many psychiatric and metabolic disorders. At that time everybody, including myself, was convinced that sugar was the culprit, and so blood sugar tests (called glucose tolerance tests or GTTs) were performed by all of us with gay abandon. Many patients did improve and, in fact, cutting out sugar, especially refined sugars and carbohydrates, was indeed a good step forward, as was reducing fat intake.

Alas! No sooner had we managed to convince our orthodox colleagues (medical doctors) that there was such a beast, we were confronted with the (at the time, unpalatable) fact that hypoglycaemia was not a disease, but only a symptom, and that the GTT was not such a good test after all. To make matters worse, in a very short time we became aware that sugar, while almost always a trigger, was neither the major nor only culprit. In fact we all learned that allergies — or intolerances as they are known — to a multitude of common foods could, and often did, cause hypoglycaemia. Once we started to test people we found hypoglycaemia caused by milk, wheat, apples and even onions! And so the era of food allergies was born! I should know — I wrote the first Australian book on the subject *(Are You Allergic to the Twentieth Century?)*.

As it turned out, nutritionists, allergists and open-minded doctors everywhere helped and cured thousands of people whose lives had become miserable because of allergies. And we are still doing it. Then a funny thing happened to some of us on the way to saving the world. We were curing thousands of people every year, yet instead of diminishing, the number of people suffering from allergies or intolerances grew, and kept growing. By pure serendipity I discovered in 1978 that some of my more recalcitrant patients were indeed suffering from an allergy to moulds–fungi (the two words are synonymous) and that one fungus, *Candida albicans,* was primarily responsible. It just so happens that this organism is the cause of a common female complaint, namely vaginal thrush (also known as monilia), an annoying but minor vaginal problem.

Around the same time, Dr Orian Truss in the United States was preparing himself to deliver to the world the concept of candida as the twentieth century scourge. This was quickly followed by Dr William Crook's now legendary book, *The Yeast Connection*. Everybody realised immediately that the *real* cause of all our problems was not hypoglycaemia or allergies at all, but actually this ubiquitous organism — the yeast fungus or *Candida albicans*. Naturally I immediately went to print with a book called *The Candida Connection in Australia,* then followed it up with *The Candida Protocol,* which was soon superseded by *The Candida Question and Answer Book*. By now I have lost count of the number of candida sufferers I have successfully treated. Many, many thousands. Suffice to say that anybody who is, or wishes to be, anybody in the alternative medicine world had to diagnose and treat candida. And thousands did, and still do. Unfortunately, some do even when candida has nothing or very little to do with the problem at hand.

Ohmygosh! Why am I, of all people, expounding such a heresy? Because shortly after the candida mania reached its peak a newfangled syndrome descended upon us, that's why! At first it was jovially known as TAT (for 'Tired All the Time' Syndrome). Then it was discovered that the syndrome was not so new after all, and in fact had been called the Post-viral Fatigue Syndrome many years before by no less an authority than the respected British medical journal *The Lancet,* only to be dismissed as a figment of the overworked imagination of some hypochrondriacs. After a while though, reports of this mysterious illness began to pour in from all over the world. Doctors being what they are, a new and far less comprehensible word was coined to define the illness — myalgic encephalomyelitis, or ME for short. The inevitable societies and self-help groups sprang into being and indeed the Australian ME Society is still called just that. This, despite the fact that there was often no muscular impairment (*myo-* means 'muscle') or inflammation to be seen and that the brain (*-cephalus*) was almost never inflamed and generally in perfectly good shape.

While many different theories were put forward by a multitude of scientists there was no general agreement as to the actual *cause* of this problem. Indeed, a school of thought existed that claimed it was a multifactorial disease. Unabated by such commonsense, the usual medical search for a single 'cause' went on. And so the era of Chronic

INTRODUCTION

Epstein Barr Virus (CEBV) Syndrome was born. This particular malaise changed names more quickly than a chameleon: EBV (for Epstein Barr Virus); Associated Fatigue Syndrome; Chronic Epstein Barr; chronic infectious mononucleosis; yuppy flu; SIDES (for Systemic Immunodeficient Epstein Barr Virus Syndrome); and finally SKIDS (which is the almost-acronym for Subclinical Immunodeficiency Syndrome). These are but a few of the names used.

It was first proposed by Dr Paul Cheney after examining 160 people in Incline, Nevada, USA. He identified four criteria with viral infections causing chronic fatigue: elevated antibodies (actually IgG VCA) to the Epstein Barr Virus; symptoms of persisting fatigue, aches and sore throats; nervous system problems like headaches, depression and difficulty concentrating; and finally, the persistence of these signs and symptoms in the absence of identifiable pathologies. If all this sounds familiar to you, it's simply because it is. Exactly the same reasons were and still are given for hypoglycaemia, allergies and candida sufferers!

During all this, I was busier than ever making the increasingly more difficult differential diagnoses between those people for whom allergies and/or candida were merely some of the *symptoms* of the Post-viral Syndrome and those for whom candida or allergies were the *primary* problem. Meanwhile we became aware that the Epstein Barr virus was not the only one causing problems and to the list of culprits we quickly added enteroviruses, cytomegalovirus (CMV), toxoplasmosis and LHV (lymphotropic herpes viruses). As the laboratory analyses of these became more available and more accurate we soon found ourselves with a whole lot of different 'causes' for the same problem.

One factor, however, remained relatively constant. In almost all cases there was some evidence of an impaired immune system and poor liver functions. Now, if one's immune system is not working properly — and it can't if the liver is not in good shape — the chances of falling victim to a viral onslaught are obviously greater than otherwise. What factor or factors, if any, were responsible for the lowered immunocompetence? In other words, why did *those* people become infected by viruses, which made them allergic and experience an explosion of candida organisms, which in turn lowered their immune efficiency even further? Two factors made some sense. The first was that the liver appeared to be implicated in most cases. The second factor was that we knew only too well that liver functions, especially critical enzymes, were easily affected by toxic chemicals.

In September 1988 there was an Australian seminar on Chronic Fatigue Syndrome chaired by authorities such as Professor John Dwyer, Andrew Lloyd, Denis Wakefield, Clem Broughton and the inimitable immunologist Robert Loblay. At the end of the seminar Dr Mark Donohoe and I took the microphone and proposed that toxic chemicals may play a significant role in Chronic Fatigue Syndrome and, by implication, in candida and allergies. Professor Dwyer was quite receptive but he explained to us that this was not his main area of research and that if we suspected chemicals had anything to do with the problem we should conduct our own studies and present it.

We did, and are still doing it. We started by taking blood samples from over 100 of our patients to the USA and having them analysed for toxic chemicals. We had to do this because the few Australian labs which offered toxic chemical tests at the time used a technique called liquid chromatography which, good as it is, can only detect these substances at levels of about 30 parts per billion. Enough for someone who is poisoned by lead or petrol fumes (say, a traffic policeman or petrol station attendant) but nowhere near enough for someone who is suffering from the effects of chronic low-grade exposure to toxic chemicals. Dr Donohoe had already told me — and the USA experts confirmed it — that we had to use a technique called gas chromatography combined with mass spectrometry with electron capture (whatever *that* means) in order to obtain meaningful results. (We can now do several of this type of test in Australia.)

While in America we took the opportunity to visit and study at Dr Bill Rea's world-famous Environmental Health Center at Dallas, Texas, where we learned the latest diagnostic, treatment and detoxification procedures. We then attended a conference at Lake Tahoe, Nevada. We listened and talked to many people. Probably the one person who crystallised the whole problem of environmental pollution and its effects on human health was Dr Stephen Levine who has written a masterpiece of a book, *Antioxidant Adaptation*.

What we have discovered from the tests, from observations and from talking to people, experts and patients alike, is that our immune systems are taking a pummelling. In our world today practically everything is a potential pollutant — the air, our food, our water supplies, our technology, our clothes and cosmetics, indeed many of the things we take for granted to make life easier. The chemical pollutants involved are well established as inducers of a variety of symptoms common to most sufferers of ecological illnesses such as allergies. Chronic infections such as *Candida albicans* or glandular fever (Epstein Barr post viral Syndrome) tend to exacerbate problems in our immune mechanisms. This is one of the reasons why chemically overloaded people or hypersensitive people are so susceptible to candida and viral illnesses. Stress, whether precipitated by emotional factors or caused by physical and chemical factors, can detrimentally affect the immune system.

During my years of clinical practice my main function has been that of diagnostician and I have often asked myself why it is that ecologically ill patients are such easy prey to infections like candida, the flu and glandular fever and why they suffer so often from chronic fatigue. It is becoming more and more evident that Dr Levine is right when he says that stress, whether chemical, physical, infectious, viral or emotional in origin can deplete our defences to the point that we suffer an increase in inflammatory, infectious and degenerative diseases.

There is no *one* cause for an illness like Chronic Fatigue Syndrome: there are many causes and each individual may have a different range of causes that produce a different range of symptoms. What we as diagnosticians must do is remain open to the possibility of a multiplicity of causes. What our patients must learn is that their doctors are not perfect. Therapists and doctors do not have all the answers. Patients have to learn to ask the right questions, just as doctors do. Mark Donohoe expresses the opinion in this book (see p. 208) that patients these days should be considered more as 'clients'.

Chronic Fatigue Syndrome is not a new illness: as I explained earlier, it has been around for quite some time but has just been known by other names. However, while it is not new, it seems to be increasing rapidly during this last part of the twentieth century. The *Journal of the American Medical Association* claimed that in May 1987 as much as 21 per cent of the general population in the United States probably had chronic immune dysfunctions. And then in March 1988 the American Academy of Otolaryngology's *Bulletin* announced that Chronic Fatigue Syndrome is potentially the most devastating disease of the twentieth century.

So, what we do know is that there is not just *one* cause of Chronic Fatigue Syndrome and also that the major problem with the syndrome is that its very complexity, its multifactorial nature, creates controversy within controversy. What I have hoped to do in *Chronic Fatigue* is cut through that complexity to explain *why* Chronic Fatigue Syndrome develops, how it is diagnosed and what you can do about it.

A Tale of Dolphins

The western portion of the Mediterranean Sea is inhabited by a beautiful type of dolphin that sports a longitudinal blue stripe along its flanks. Appropriately called 'striped dolphins', these gentle mammals are often washed ashore — dead for one reason or another — at a rate of approximately 50 per year.

In mid 1990, more than 50 dead dolphins were washed ashore on the French coast in one 14-day period alone. The same year, on the Spanish coast, the count was 250 dead dolphins in less than three months. The official cause of death? The same virus that causes human measles.

Not new to viral deaths, marine inhabitants have been decimated by viral epidemics during the past decade. In 1988 some twenty thousand seals were killed by one particular virus. Of course, this used to happen to humans. The world's population has been subjected to one epidemic or another for millennia. What makes this latest example of aquatic mayhem different to anything that has previously occurred on earth — and terribly important to our understanding of modern humans' health — is the fact that when the poor dolphins were examined, autopsies showed their tissues were contaminated with heavy metals and PCBs (polychlorinated biphenyls). The implication is that these xenobiotics (toxic foreign chemicals) weakened the dolphins' immune systems, making them vulnerable to viral attacks. And so it is with humans.

Our Bodies – Our Environment

Environmental Medicine and Total Load

There is little doubt the environment is at fault in the majority of human illnesses in general, and chronic fatigue in particular, but it depends on one's definition of the word 'environment'. If we mean the colloquial understanding of the word in all its variety (ozone, greenhouse, chemical, air pollution, etc.), then the environment is NOT always the cause. But if we mean 'the total sum of everything hereditary, physical (viral, bacterial, etc.), psychological and personal to which we are exposed', then by this definition we can claim that ALL illnesses, whether physical, psychological, bacterial or viral, are really environmental illnesses. The use of the word 'environment' therefore, when we talk about illness doesn't mean the environment as a whole (the earth, the atmosphere, the ecosystems, and so on), but rather the *immediate* environment of an individual.

A virus is less likely to make us very ill if we are happy, well nourished and not full of chemicals. On the other hand, if we are under a viral attack, we may well become so delicate that even a relatively small amount of a common chemical will make us sick.

So what is to blame? The chemical or the virus? And what about our general health BEFORE we were struck by the virus or exposed to the chemicals?

We are the first generation of human beings to be exposed to an unprecedented number of chemicals.

We are the first generation to tighten/insulate our buildings so that the quality of the indoor environment is often worse than that of the outside fresh air.

We are also the first generation to eat a diet high in refined carbohydrates, tinned foods, takeaway fast meals and foods whose nutrients have been cooked or processed out of them.

We are the first generation to be exposed to a magnitude of electromagnetic radiations.

We are more sedentary than ever and we are bombarded by an ever-increasing amount of sensory inputs and information that we have difficulty processing.

We are also assailed by stresses we have no practical recourse against in the sense that we can't 'fight or flight' them as our cave-dwelling ancestors could when confronted by a threat.

We are reaching a point now where our capacity to detoxify, in all ways, is no longer equal to the magnitude of inputs.

In a real sense then, the new medicine is *environmental* medicine. Its most basic principle is that of TOTAL LOAD, which simply means that whatever affects our daily lives may slowly accumulate. If our load is light we can probably shrug off or fight almost any stress, bacteria or virus that assails us. If the load is excessive, our ability to cope is reduced and we run the risk of losing our health. Once lost, it is somewhat pointless to look for a single 'cause' for our illness, as it may well be that the total, cumulative weight of the 'load' makes it impossible to get well, no matter what single symptom or disease we direct our forces against.

One way to help you understand this very important principle is to tell you a tale.

Two people were standing on a steep road which climbed to a village high up on a hill. Halfway along the road there was a mule attached to a cart full of bulging, coloured bags. The mule had stopped because it could not pull the load any further. The cart was just too heavy.

The two well-meaning people felt sorry for the mule and wanted to help. They first discussed what medicine they could administer to the mule to give it more strength. When they couldn't think of anything suitable they decided to help the mule by taking some of the load off the cart.

They began to argue about which bag should be taken off first. They had different opinions. One thought the bright red bags should go first because they looked *heavy*. The other favoured the brown ones because they looked *bigger*. So they argued. And the donkey stood still, patiently exhausted. A wise old man who lived in the village on top of the hill happened by the scene. After listening for a few minutes, the wise old man approached the cart and, with never a word, started to throw off whatever bag he could get hold of. After a while the mule sensed the new lightness of the load and resumed his climb. The wise old man then turned to the onlookers and said: 'I appreciate your good intentions but none of us can see inside the bags; hence we don't know if the big brown ones are full of feathers — or lead. The red ones look ominous, but they may be full of leaves — or bricks. I knew I could never take off ALL the bags, so I just took off as many as I could. I knew that if I kept on reducing the *total load*, the mule would eventually be able to pull the cart along.'

That is how every therapist should approach illness.

The Immune System

One day, a long time ago, I was watching in fascination while one of my children spent what seemed an interminable time (and quite a few dollars) playing PAC MAN (a computer game similar to Space Invaders) and I started to think about our immune system. Believe me, what happens on the electronic game table is remarkably similar to the events which take place when our natural defences (in the immune system) try to protect us from germs, viruses, bacteria and other 'enemies' that are lurking around waiting, as it were, to zap our health. The scenario would do justice to Steven Spielberg. In fact it could well be called the 'Inner Star Wars'. Or how about *Bloodstream Galactica*? Sound fantastic? Well, just to drive the point home, here is the inner star wars plan:

Just as there are different forces, different ranks and different areas of activity in an army, so it happens in your immune system. This is the way it works:

1. An enemy enters the body and starts to multiply.
2. Neutrophils and natural killer cells on patrol try to destroy the enemy.

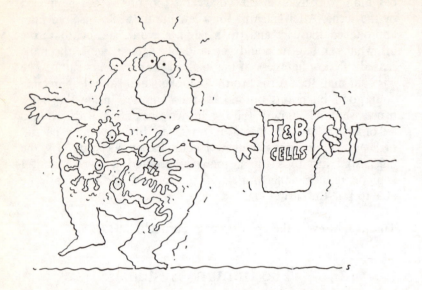

3 A group of proteins known as 'complements' mark the invaders for recognition by some of the immune army.
4 Macrophages sound the alarm bell and send messages to the T helper cells.
5 T helpers activate the armed forces.
6 B cells make antibodies against certain specific enemies.
7 Antibodies disarm the invaders and stimulate the complements to do their work.
8 Killer T cells destroy cancer and virus-infected cells.
9 Suppressor T cells slow down, or stop, the immune response before it goes haywire and starts to attack itself and the host's body (autoimmune disease).
10 Some of the T and B cells are trained to recognise the enemy and attack immediately should they appear again.

Non-specific immunity is an immediate reaction by one cell to a variety of enemies.

Specific immunity is a process in which one specific cell attacks a particular enemy. It is usually a delayed reaction.

Cell-mediated immunity is a process in which T cells patrol the body and destroy abnormal cells before they have a chance to multiply. They also help regulate the work of the immune army.

Human beings, like most other organisms, live in a largely hostile environment, surrounded by an incredible array of bacteria, viruses, parasites, mycotoxins and other assorted 'bugs' whose main aim in life seems to be the destruction of law-abiding citizens who are peacefully going about their business. As if an abundant supply of 'natural' enemies such as staphylococci, chlamydia, retroviruses, lentoviruses, *Candida albicans,* and more wasn't enough, we have spent the last 100 years or so adding a cornucopia of human-made chemicals to our water, air and food — in other words to our environment. All these, whether natural or artificial, can become enemies; they are known as *antigens*.

The ability to distinguish what belongs to the body and what does not applies to a lot more than just potentially harmful micro-organisms and chemicals. The immune system will cause a body to reject even perfectly normal proteins if they originate from 'outside'.

When we eat 'foreign' proteins, such as animal meats, these have to be first broken down to single amino acids. This is achieved by special enzymes in the digestive tract. Only then can these proteins, now in fragments, be absorbed. At this stage they are no longer real proteins, but only their constituents. These constituent proteins are the same in all animals, so they are not foreign or threatening. The body then uses these building blocks to re-synthesise its own proteins to repair or create whatever it needs. The final product is unique to that body only.

We all know, for example, that transplanting organs between people is not very easy. One of the major problems is rejection. Our immune system tends to reject even cells from other individuals of the same species, unless they are identical to those of its own body.

We all encounter an enormous variety of antigens or potential enemies every day of our lives. In addition to micro-organisms, antigens can be drugs, animal venoms, insect bites, foods, and so on. So, an efficient immune system must include defenders (lymphocytes) which can recognise every single antigen we are likely to meet in a lifetime. What a tall order! And one that is becoming increasingly difficult when we remember that we are dumping thousands of new chemicals into our environment every single year. Even without these, an immune system capable of lasting a few decades means that millions of different lymphocyte receptors must be able to recognise just about every antigen found in nature or created in a laboratory! If the immune system is not capable of recognising an antigen, then the substance may become toxic, even lethal. It stands to reason that an incompetent immune system will not protect us very well. Perhaps when we most need it.

As a shrewd observer once noted, if germs were meant to kill us, the first epidemic would have wiped out humankind. But it didn't (not so far, anyway!). The reason is quite simple. The police, army, navy and air forces within us somehow managed to protect *some* people, allowing the human race to continue to proliferate. During the early biological catastrophes, such as the Black Plague, we hardly had doctors worthy of the name, let alone antibiotics or hospitals; yet many survived. The only reason they did is that some of us possess a great deal of resistance.

The human body is eminently capable of defending and even healing itself. As Dr Ronald Glasser once said:

> To cure a disease, not just to treat it, you must help the body to do it itself. It is the body that is the hero, not science, not antibiotics nor machines or new devices. It is the body making antibodies against the swallowed polio vaccine, not the iron lung, that cures polio. It is the body, not radiation or drugs, that must destroy cancer cells if the patient is to survive.

Pasteur, the father of the germ theory, once said that it was not bacteria but the 'soil' on which it fell that made all the difference between health and disease. What he meant, of course, was that although we are constantly inhaling, ingesting and touching germs of all kinds, only relatively few of these organisms will actually manage to cause us any harm. You can sow seeds all you like; if the ground is not receptive, you'll grow nothing!

It is pretty clear that for anything to affect us to any degree we must, at the time, be weak enough for the 'enemy' to be able to overcome us. Our ability to resist anything is often called our general resistance. Scientists define this as our immunocompetence.

HOW THE IMMUNE SYSTEM WORKS

There are two basic components of the immune system:

Natural immunity consists primarily of physical and some chemical barriers. They include skin secretions, sweat and tears, mucus, and an array of enzymes in the digestive, respiratory and urinary tracts.

Acquired immunity consists of a large 'army' of fighters, each with a special capacity.

The most common cells of our immune system are the *granulocytes,* of which there are three types: *neutrophils, oesinophils* and *basophils*. They are the ones we check first, with a blood test, to ascertain if a bacterial infection or an allergy is present.

Then there are the *lymphocytes*. The two main types of lymphocytes are the *B cells* and the *T cells*. There are several kinds of T cells. All lymphocytes look alike and special tests are needed to differentiate them. Counting the different types of lymphocytes helps in the evaluation of immune deficiencies or disruptions. Lymphocyte counts are important warning signs for diseases such as cancer, AIDS and autoimmune diseases.

Then there are the *monocytes* and the *macrophages*. They are the scavengers of our immunity — the garbage collectors. They eat up sick cells that are about to die and scavenge any foreign material they find.

The neutrophils attack bacteria vigorously but they do so in a sort of suicide mission. Like Kamikaze pilots, they hurl themselves onto bacteria and engulf them and usually die in the process. The bacteria is actually killed by hydrogen peroxide produced, and then released, by neutrophils at the site. After it's all over, the pus you see is what remains of all the dead neutrophils.

Oesinophils, by contrast, tend to come on strongly when there are allergies or some type of infection, especially by parasites. It does not matter whether the allergy shows up as eczema or asthma, oesinophils are asked to get to work.

The lymphocytes are another matter altogether. B lymphocytes produce antibodies. Actually they are first carried on the cell surface and at that stage are called immunoglobulins. When they are released into the body's fluids they become antibodies. These are specialised proteins that can attach themselves to foreign molecules, such as bacteria, the outer coats of viruses, etc. Every B cell has the capacity to produce a great number of its own special antibody, but refrains from doing so until these are needed. Once immunoglobulins bind to an antigen, B cells can start dividing rapidly and begin to produce plasma cells. One plasma cell can then make some 2000 antibody molecules EACH SECOND.

The T cells aid and abet the B cells in their chores. Just like a type of smell or perfume can turn someone on while an unpleasant odour may turn them off, so the T cells turn B cells on or off. One type, known as helpers or T4 cells, turns the B cells on while another, called suppressor or T8 cells, turns the B cells off whenever there are already enough antibodies. A sort of 'cease production' order. They are the brakes of the immune system.

All sorts of things can affect various parts of the immune system. Malnutrition and starvation tend to lower T cell numbers, especially T4s, or can cause them to malfunction. Chemicals (xenobiotics) tend to alter T cell ratios and suppress T4s. Others affect a group of cells called natural killers (NKs) or the T4:T8 ratio. Other xenobiotics can affect the thymic epithelium, B cell differentiation, T cell regulation, macrophage functions, protein synthesis and B cell functions.

Many drugs can affect immunity. The effects of aspirin on granulocytes, for example, is well documented. Toxins from various fungi and several from *Candida albicans* can affect some components of the immune system. On the other hand, some infections are difficult to treat and tend to recur more frequently when blood sugar levels are elevated. So even a simple dietary manipulation, like eating less sugar (and that, I am afraid, includes fructose, as in fruit juices) can affect our immunity.

In reality, the matter is far more complicated than the above simplified explanation. There are other essential components, such as antigen presenting cells (APCs) and the major histocompatibility complex (MHC).

Another group of T lymphocytes, known as cytotoxic cells, act as professional assassins. They kill the cell outright. Their main targets are body cells infected with viruses which they destroy before the virus proliferates. The same cells are also part of our defence against cancer.

Another problem is overstimulation, usually associated with not enough T suppressor cells, which causes some cells of the immune system to go on a rampage, attacking everything in sight. The result of this includes inflammation and such diseases as Hashimoto's thyroiditis, multiple sclerosis, lupus, SLE, autoimmune encephalomyelitis, and rheumatoid and adjuvant arthritis.

WHAT DISRUPTS THE IMMUNE SYSTEM?
Unfortunately many well-meaning, but ill-informed people think that the only problem with CFS is a reduced activity of the immune system. Alas! This is clearly not so. First of all, blood tests of people suffering from chronic fatigue often show some parts of one's immunity are down, while others are overactive. Then there is the constant spectre of autoimmune diseases — those illnesses that are caused by EXCESSIVE activity of the immune system.

Autoimmunity, in which the immune system recognises and attacks the body's own tissues, is not as simple as it once seemed. The ability to self-recognise appears to be at the heart of health as well as certain diseases. In addition, the immune system can be affected in ways that cause it to over-respond one day, and under-respond another.

Be that as it may, let us look at what can alter immune functions by making them operate in ways that can cause poor health, and, in some cases, CFS.

Poor nutrition
This is one of the most frequent causes of immunodeficiency.

Disrupted natural immunity
The physical barrier of our natural immunity can be affected by simple factors like cuts of the skin, lack of protective (waxy) coating on the skin, insufficient mucus secretions, etc.

Viral infections
Once it was believed that only severe viral infections affected our immunity. I have seen many a patient who has received advice from one practitioner or another who suggested that, in the absence of a previous viral infection, CFS, if a valid diagnosis at all, MUST be of other origin — usually chemical.

Such ignorance, however, is very forgivable. It is not so much a matter of ignorance as one of time and experience.

Be that as it may, when someone does NOT get well, or when progress is too slow, or when it is marred by excessive and frequent relapses, one must consider the usefulness of recent advances in medical knowledge. One such advance is that we now know that it is quite possible to suffer with all sorts of disease, including CFS, from a virus which entered our body years, even decades, before and has done so without provoking, at the time, any significant symptoms.

These viruses, generally known as latent viruses or, in special cases, slow viruses, can and do affect our immunity in several, and often quite damaging, ways. In addition, there are some seventy-four varieties of enterovirus, each of which can cause CFS-like illnesses.

Fortunately there are now at least some tests that help hard working diagnosticians like myself find out when this is the case.

Keeping up anti-viral measures is always a good way to prevent, as well as treat, any kind of viral infection.

Vaccination
This is a very controversial subject but, in the opinion of many scientists, vaccination can affect our immunity in many ways.

Drugs
Many, if not most, drugs, alter immune functions, especially steroids.

Xenobiotics (toxic chemicals)
These can have dramatic effects on the immune system. In fact, ALL chemicals must be suspect. The pertinent questions are: Which chemical (because each has a different action)? What amount? Over what period of time? In combination with which other factors?

Stress
This is, without doubt, an important factor in triggering, precipitating and aggravating CFS. Unfortunately, what is stressful to one individual may just be 'water off a duck's back' to another. Also, the same individual may find that one event, situation or factor is stressful at one time, but not at another time.

In general, stress does not 'cause' illness as such. It can, however, 'unmask' an existing condition or aggravate an underlying situation so its effects become manifest. CFS patients have a very low tolerance for stress of any kind, hence the need to differentiate between various types of CFS as well as different types of stress.

Temperature

Temperature changes, especially the cold, tend to aggravate viral CFS and some of its symptoms. The same is not always true with chemical CFS because there seem to be so many individual variations.

WHAT CAN WE DO TO HELP OR PROTECT OUR IMMUNITY?

'Mummy, I feel sick — it hurts,' cries the child pointing to the abdomen, or head, or chest. With an almost Pavlovian reflex you, a good parent, will take the child's temperature and, if it's high, make an anguished call to the doctor, who may prescribe aspirin or another fever-reducing medicine. Perhaps you may administer one yourself, from whatever you can find in the bathroom cabinet. You may be making a big mistake!

Yesterday's knowledge becomes today's heresy and tomorrow's dogma. In no area is this more prevalent than in the science and art of medicine. From blood-letting to Pasteur, from herbalism to acupuncture, we have seen old truths revived, new theories fought tooth-and-nail by doctors, and medical opinion constantly reversed. One of the most glaring examples is the popular (and scientific) attitude to high body temperatures.

Your eyes ache, your muscles are sore, your joints feel stiff, and you are perspiring. You take your temperature and it turns out to be 40°C (104°F); so you decide to be your own doctor and take a couple of aspirins — to bring the temperature down, of course.

Until one hundred years ago some doctors were inducing fever in patients as a treatment for various illnesses, even cancer (a procedure which is today again being used experimentally by a few researchers). However, this attitude to fever came to an abrupt halt at the beginning of this century with the advent of aspirin. People began to associate the drug's ability to alleviate aches and pains with the fact that almost invariably there was a reduction in the patient's temperature. Unable, or unwilling to think laterally, doctors and patients alike decided fever was an 'enemy'.

By 1969 Nobel Prize laureate Andre Wolff began to question

the dogma that fever should be attacked. He theorised that if a physiological response to illness has remained with us for millions of years, it must serve some useful purpose. Working at the Pasteur Institute in Paris, he discovered that the polio virus did not thrive when its surrounding temperature approached 40°C (104°F). At temperatures between 38.5°C (101.3°F) and 39°C (102.2°F) he found that the infectious ability of the virus could be reduced by more than 90 per cent, which means that even a slight elevation in temperature has at least some effect in beginning to inhibit viruses.

By 1975 physiologist Mathew Kluger, then at the University of Michigan Medical School, noted that although the elevation of temperature which normally goes hand-in-hand with many diseases was observed, noted and studied for hundreds of years, no-one had ever convincingly established that it was harmful.

In 1977 James Fruthaler, Clinical Professor of Paediatrics at Tulane University in the United States, declared that: 'Since the height of a fever is not important, there is no need to take [children's] temperature routinely.' He had searched the literature (he said this in 1984) again and again, and could not find '. . . a single case of brain damage due to high fever unless the disease that caused the fever, such as encephalitis or meningitis, also caused brain damage'.

In 1979, one of the world's most important scientific journals, *Science,* reported Kluger and his colleague, B. Rothenburg, saying that: 'Doctors' eagerness to prescribe drugs like aspirin to bring down a fever may do more harm than good'.

As research proceeded during the 1980s Patrick Murphy, of the prestigious Johns Hopkins University School of Medicine, said that 'People who think, nowadays think of fever as a protective mechanism for the body, instead of a harmful one.' This abrupt (for medicine) change of heart is primarily due to a series of remarkably simple observations and experiments by Kluger. Kluger took some animals and made them sick: those which developed a fever survived, those which did not, died. Since these experiments, researchers have found similar effects in humans and we are beginning to unravel the mechanics of fever.

The temperature of humans is kept within fairly narrow limits. A drop below 25°C (77°F) or a rise above 45°C (113°F) for anything but a short time is usually fatal. A portion of the brain known as the hypothalamus is responsible for policing the limited range and it works very much like the thermostat in an air-conditioner. Fever occurs when the thermostat in the brain is turned up, usually in response to infections, but occasionally as a result of allergic or rheumatic illnesses. An endogenous pyrogen (EP), by the name of hormone interlukin-1, is released from white blood cells when a foreign substance enters the blood stream. That is why temperature may rise during an allergic reaction or in some rheumatic autoimmune diseases. Of course, it is therefore released by the body in response to bacterial or viral attacks and it actually seeks out the temperature-controlling centre within the brain (hypothalamus), causing in turn the release of another hormone, prostaglandin, which tells the brain's thermostat to 'set' temperatures at a much higher level. Just like a furnace, the body generates additional heat (by burning fats and causing shivering), and the higher temperature activates the immune system.

Researchers at Yale University have shown that fever and interlukin-1 can increase the production of T-lymphocyte cells and disease-fighting antibodies up to 20 times, while the effectiveness of the anti-viral agent interferon is greatly increased. Dr Kluger and his associates also noted that as the temperature of infected animals begins to rise, their levels of iron fall in their blood. Any decrease in iron levels makes it more difficult for bacteria to survive and multiply. During some of Kluger's experiments he noted that 'infected lizards given iron supplements were more likely to die than those who were not given any supplements of that mineral'.

In another way old folk wisdom seems to have come up trumps. Egg-white was sometimes used on open wounds and scratches on the skin. Egg-white contains conalbumin, a substance which binds iron, so the micro-organisms can't use it to proliferate. In the fight against infections, especially viral ones, one of the most important factors is an ample supply of ascorbic acid (the more acid, the more effective it is against viruses) and some, but not too much, zinc, which is well-known for its ability to antagonise and displace iron. At the same time I have found that the milder forms of vitamin C, such as calcium ascorbate and other more alkaline forms of this vitamin, are far less effective, and sometimes downright counter-productive in the treatment of infectious diseases, partly because they are more alkaline (bacteria hate acidity but thrive in alkalinity), and partly because excessive calcium may decrease the absorption of zinc from the digestive system. This in turn can cause difficulties in utilising magnesium and pyridoxine (vitamin B6), which also play an important role in the functioning of our immune system.

Concerned parents *do* have a legitimate fear of fever-induced convulsions — they do occur, but they are far less common than you may believe. Available statistics show that the rate among pre-school children is less than three per cent, and even lower in older children. Temperatures around, or above 42°C (102-103°F) can, however, be dangerous during pregnancy if they are sustained, and they can increase the heart rate by about ten beats per minute for each degree (Fahrenheit) above normal, thus posing a threat for patients with cardiovascular disease. Very high temperatures may also aggravate underlying conditions and, because they increase the body's demands for oxygen, may pose a serious strain on patients with respiratory illnesses.

Recently, publicity has been given to a technique which involves the heating of AIDS patients' blood. This apparently cures or at least greatly improves the condition of the sufferers. The AIDS virus is, in some respects, similar to the ones that can cause CFS.

Doctors are in the business of making people feel better. But now that we know that patients precluded from having a fever can deteriorate, or recover more slowly, it is difficult to understand why doctors, and some parents, insist on giving fever-suppressing drugs as soon as there is a rise in body temperature.

Mucus

In the respiratory tract, the first line of defence is the small hairs (nasal cilia) which trap some particles from the air we breathe. The mucus then catches more foreign matter and keeps it away from the actual cells. Macrophages along the tract take care of them. If the material is expelled through coughing or spitting, that's that. What is swallowed ends up in the next protection trap: the digestive system. The stomach is very hostile to foreign matter. Its acidity kills and destroys just about anything.

When we get a cold or flu, the body reacts by producing a lot of mucus. Many of the invading viruses are eliminated through the mucus. It is therefore not really a good idea to reach for the cold and flu tablets the minute you get sick. The decongestants built into them to dry up the mucus secretions take away one of the body's lines of defence. These preparations also contain a cocktail of other chemicals that merely add to the load of chemicals our bodies have to deal with.

Gut flora

An organism that invades our digestive tract will find the competition with the residents is fierce and that the gut flora is even capable of making its own antibiotics. That is why you will read so often that the treatment of malfunctions of the digestive system causing *dysbiosis* (which simply means an abnormal rate or ratio of intestinal bugs that make up the gut flora) is important, even critical, to the treatment of intestinal thrush (candida) and other factors associated with CFS.

In this, various types of *Lactobacillus acidophilus,* garlic and other vitamins and minerals are of great help in helping to re-establish the proper balance between useful and dangerous gut residents. It is also one reason why antibiotics (useful only to combat bacteria, not viruses or chemicals) can actually make matters worse. Pharmaceutical antibiotics tend to destroy the good inhabitants of the gut, along with a few 'enemies'. Generally, they tend to further unbalance the ratio between them and, in addition, they often suppress immune activity.

The urinary and reproductive tracts tend to offer some protection by the acidity of their fluids and the presence of a type of enzyme known as *lysosome.* Also found in tears, this enzyme kills some bacteria.

Anti-oxidants and free radical scavengers

Boosting these factors almost invariably will help CFS patients. The types, quantities and ratios of these and many vitamins, minerals and other supplements vary dramatically with the type of CFS treated (viral CFS or chemical CFS) and with the individual.

In addition, the treatment of each of the major 'symptoms' may require the use of some specific supplement while rendering others inappropriate and, in some cases, counterproductive.

Be guided by your practitioner.

Exercise

The main casualties of the fitness craze may well be CFS sufferers, especially those with an underlying viral problem. And for those with a xenobiotics problem, jogging is not only counter-productive, but often very dangerous. In general though it very much depends on what kind of exercise for what kind of CFS.

Strenuous exercise tends to lower immune functions, making it contraindicated in practically all cases of CFS. Jogging can cause an increased inhalation of pollutants and an increase in lactic acid. The first is obviously not helpful; the second would aggravate Lactate Induced Anxiety Syndrome (LIAS).

Additionally, gyms often use powerful disinfectants and cleansing materials that release fumes for a long time after they are applied. Strenuous gym work-outs may cause problems in chemically sensitive or already overloaded individuals.

In the past few years we have seen not only a large increase in the number of people treated for exercise-related musculo-skeletal problems but also an increased incidence of some of the factors, such as Epstein Barr virus, closely associated with CFS. In fact, some researchers are beginning to suggest that one of the many possible reasons why there has been such an accelerated rise in the number of CFS sufferers may well be the huge increase in exercise fanatics.

Strenuous exercise does increase the output of certain hormones and brain chemicals to which one can become addicted. What is sometimes not understood is that withdrawal from these, such as must occur whenever one is NOT exercising, may affect our immunity.

On the other hand, some forms of gentle exercise, especially certain types of yoga or Tai Chi, can be quite helpful. People with an underlying chemical problem can, under some special circumstances, benefit from exercise.

Relaxation, meditation and general rest are almost invariably more helpful than exercise for people who are ill. This applies even more so to CFS sufferers.

Gamma globulin (GG)

Injections and drips of GG have been very useful with some people. The problem is that, at the time of writing, practically all the physicians who have used it agree that the effects of GG can be very unpredictable. It is most used on viral CFS patients, when the liver has been affected, and in these cases it is either very helpful, sometimes very quickly, or it is of no help at all. In chemical CFS the positive results are far less encouraging and so we seldom use it in treating such cases these days.

Toxic chemicals

If you suspect that toxic chemicals in your environment are causing you ill health or CFS, then one course of action could be to remove oneself from the chemicals by selling your house and moving into another one that has been specially constructed to be free of these chemicals.

This is not practicable for most people, and a better course of action might be to consult a therapist who will investigate your condition. The therapist may decide to boost your immunity with diet, supplements, etc., and arrange for levels of chemicals and antigens in your environment to be checked and taken care of, and treat the underlying things that have weakened you, such as allergies, candida, viruses.

Stress

There is little doubt that stress can aggravate almost any problem. On the other hand a little stress of the right kind has actually been found to BOOST immunity! Often it is not a matter of the stress itself, but the way an individual REACTS to the stress that makes the difference.

So, psychology, counselling, emotional support and plenty of old-fashioned TLC are a very good, even essential medicine!

Diets, vitamins, minerals, amino acids and other supplements

Special remedies such as echinacea and some homeopathic medicines are invaluable in the fight against CFS, but again, they have to be prescribed individually. That is one reason why, apart from a general elimination diet and a particular candida diet, you will not find in this book a set prescription for treatment. Let me make that quite clear. What helps one person may not help you. It could perhaps even harm you. After all, you would not wear anyone else's denture, or bra, or glasses.

Further, there is a more subtle, and therefore more worrying, danger. Some supplements or medicines that are useful in some cases, are not so in another type of CFS or are only contraindicated *at some stage* of the treatment but not another. Biotin and cysteine are such supplements.

Iron supplements can make progress months, even years longer. Taking some types of vitamin C such as calcium ascorbate in very large doses can actually wipe out any progress for weeks on end. Bonemeal preparations may be contaminated with lead.

We have already seen the possible dangers of excessively low cholesterol regimens.

Advice you will often hear is to eat plenty of fresh fruit and vegetables. Alas! Some unfortunate individuals are affected by natural chemicals contained in many of them (solanine in tomatoes and potatoes, salicylates in apples and avocado, etc.) Some people are allergic to gluten (wheat, rye, buckwheat, malt, barley). Fruit juices, apart from the fact that they may cause blood sugar and therefore cellular ageing if taken on an empty stomach, can actually CAUSE a flare up of intestinal thrush that can cause a relapse or put the CFS treatment program back for months.

Another popular advice, again, usually given by well-meaning individuals with little or no clinical experience, is to 'listen to your body'; to eat and drink what makes you feel better. The problem here is that the body of a CFS sufferer may not be able to give the right signals. Often, in fact, it gives distorted, quite unreliable signals which are easily misunderstood. Sweets and cakes make many, perhaps most, people feel better. It does not mean they are good for you. If your blood sugar is low, a few tablespoons of sugar will fix it. But you will pay for it as soon as the blood sugar levels start to fall, giving you the symptoms of hypoglycaemia. Any drug addict will tell you how much better it feels after taking a dose and how unwell one can be when not having one handy.

I advise many, but not all, of my patients NOT to listen to their body until they are well again.

Biochemical Individuality

In the province of Northern Sonora, Mexico, there lives a tribe of Indians by the name of Tarahumara which has been the subject of much medical research because they can run some 50 kilometres per day in very high altitudes, and do this day after day.

When doctors tested one runner just after he arrived back from one such run, they found his heartbeat was slower than when he began. Yet the Indians live mainly on corn and a few root vegetables. One of the most sub-standard nutritional regimens possible and one that is notorious for causing many health problems such as pellagra. Apparently these Indians are able not only to remain healthy, which is extraordinary enough, but can perform incredible feats of endurance.

When placed on a nutritionally balanced diet, with vitamins, minerals and other nutritional supplements, many become quite ill. They develop heart disease, high blood pressure and skin problems.

As Hippocrates said: 'Some can eat their fill of cheese without any unpleasant consequences, and those whom it suits are wonderfully strengthened by it . . . [Others] have something in the body which is inimical to cheese and this is aroused and disturbed by it.'

In other words, 'One man's meat is another man's poison.' But how often, today, do we utter this hallowed phrase about anything and everything but food? Whether we're vegetarians or steak 'n' salad freaks, Pritikin followers or Atkins advocates, we feel our way is right.

But right for whom?

Modern medical science calls this personalised reaction to food *biochemical individuality*. Hippocrates knew it well. But the man who expounded this principle in modern times (seeing that all great principles need expounding every few centuries) was Dr Roger Williams, of the University of Texas — a biochemist. Dr Williams, who incidentally discovered pantothenic acid or vitamin B5, wrote an excellent book on the subject, appropriately called *You Are Unique*.

In this book Dr Williams explains that, firstly, our anatomy is unique. It's not just our faces and fingerprints; our hearts, lungs and livers don't look the same either, and often not remotely like the organs that appear in medical textbooks. Variations in other parts of the human anatomy are obvious.

So each of us is different — and nowhere more different than in our ideas about what is desirable food. But our bodies may have other ideas; and even 100 per cent natural food may provoke strong resistance in an unwilling body. We all know, for instance, people with allergies to pineapples, lobsters, tomatoes, and citrus fruits — even to sunshine, if the person happens to be albino. The cause? Biochemical individuality.

This means there's really no such thing as a 'good' food or

a 'bad' one. Each one of us ingests large amounts of chemicals — additives, colourants, preservatives and so on — in our daily diet; and while many of us show no visible ill-effects others are made very ill indeed by these things.

THE MYTH OF 'RECOMMENDED DAILY ALLOWANCES'

Why then should we be surprised to learn that some people may need twice, or more, the recommended daily allowance of a particular vitamin to remain healthy? Recommended allowance for what day? The day they fire you and you come home in bumper-to-bumper traffic to find your spouse has run off with the yoga teacher and your dog has turned rabid? Or the first day of your vacation when you're lying in lush grass under a shady willow listening to babbling brooks and birds?

Sometimes our greater need for a vitamin, mineral or certain biochemical substance, is just a passing thing. Because, say, we've moved to a colder climate for six months, or we've flown halfway around the world on urgent business, or it's the stress of exams, getting divorced, having a parent die or having a virus take up residence in our upper respiratory tract.

But while it's true to say the 'average' person can exist on 50 milligrams of vitamin C per day, or on 40-50 grams of protein per day (barring emergency situations like those above), there are also people, who, to function normally, just need more (or less) of some substance all the time. This is what's called vitamin dependency, as opposed to vitamin deficiency.

So it's crazy, isn't it, to say people should eat more protein, or less fat, or more soya beans and definitely never touch seaweed? We're all different.

WHY ARE THERE MORE SENSITIVE PEOPLE TODAY?

It's true doctors are on the look-out earlier, and are therefore better able to pick up lots of things. But we must also consider how great-grandmother lived. A hundred or so years ago, and especially in the country, a pregnant woman wasn't exposed to the medicinal drugs and chemicalised foodstuffs we have today. Hence, her unborn baby may have got a better start — if it didn't die at birth or in the early months. Only the tough survived. Now, with greater hospitalisation of maternity cases, better sanitation and the success in controlling infectious diseases like cholera and diphtheria, more and more babies make it — perhaps by the skin of their teeth. And they in turn have babies, who inherit the weaknesses.

Hence, the number of people born with these errors of metabolism, with suspect enzymes, is likely to increase even further. And, meanwhile, there are more hazards in our food, our water, and our environment every day. In fact, it's often impossible to know what's in our food.

So although the human body can cope and adjust wonderfully in many ways, the day of reckoning finally comes. Scientists know it's never JUST the last straw that breaks the camel's back. The crisis comes from the cumulative, synergistic effect of many separate stresses — dietary, environmental, emotional factors working together until one day the body cries, 'I've had enough!'

MUTATION
There is a substantial body of scientific evidence that constant bombardment from atomic radiation and exposure to an increasing number of chemicals are mutating our genes.

Recent work done by Dr Barry Commoner shows that the longer one cooks food, say a hamburger, the more mutagens are produced. Similarly, any process which involves lengthy boiling, as in the extraction of yeast spreads from vegetable/cereal substances, also creates mutagens.

ENZYMES
We inherit our enzymes from our forebears — sometimes directly from our parents, sometimes indirectly through our parents from an earlier ancestor.

Biochemical individuality is largely a result of enzymes. Some individuals have faulty enzymes, some are lacking specific enzymes, etc. The classic definition says that an 'enzyme' is a catalyst, that is, something that can change substance A into substance B while remaining unchanged itself. For instance, yeast is a catalyst because a little bit of yeasty dough can be used to turn more flour and water into a second loaf of bread. Yogurt is a catalyst because with a little bit you can turn milk into more yogurt. But custard is not a catalyst because it won't turn milk into more custard.

This makes it sound as though enzymes can last a long time, endlessly creating miracles. They can — but only if they're treated with respect. Enzymes are fragile things. Excessive heat makes them bounce and shake loose from their foundations; incorrect acidity or alkalinity kills them. So how, then, do enzymes survive inside the human body, when its acid/alkaline balance, or pH, shifts from the neutral figure of 7.0, or when we run a temperature of 40°C (104°F)?

Enzymes break down, or sign themselves off, all the time. But they are replaced constantly, because inside each of our cells, in the nucleus, is the DNA molecule which holds the vital recipe for your own, individualised, enzyme. If it's wrong to start with, at the time of conception, then it's likely to stay wrong most of your life. The body seldom has second thoughts, and finds it difficult to make adjustments with enzymes. When it does, it may take a long time — perhaps a longer time than you've got.

Enzymes are also destroyed, and very quickly too, by poisons. For example, cyanide. Other poisons, less terminal, can nevertheless affect and mutate your enzymes so sneakily that you just don't realise what's happening. This is one way, and a not very nice one, that your enzymes can change.

The job of enzymes is to combine with incoming foodstuffs and turn, say a piece of steak, into minute particles of slush (amino acids, lipids, carbohydrates) that can be squeezed through the outer wall of the cells to provide nourishment. Altogether the body contains millions of enzymes, which function in systems and are strung out in certain pathways, like signals along a railway line. If one breaks down, or is erratic or missing, chaos can result.

Fortunately, vitamins, minerals and a proper hormone balance can do a lot to make so-so enzyme systems more efficient.

DIET

More radiation, more drugs, more pollution, more chemicals in our food: it's not surprising that today a biochemical chink in our armour can spell trouble.

But the biggest stress to our body's myriad enzymatic processes is food — because that's what keeps coming at us three times a day, or even more often, from the day we're born.

For most of the human race's life on earth the only problem about food was getting enough of it. For twelve hours a day or more, men hunted animals and women searched for eggs, berries and nuts, and once food got past the teeth there wasn't much to worry about. No great detective work was necessary to trace a violent tummy-ache, or sudden death, to the new fruit or seed the whole village had seen you eat the day before.

But today the effect of our food is much more subtle, as we'll see. It's not a matter of life and death so much as years of feeling below par and never quite knowing why. You may never connect the fact that your headaches come before your breakfast grapefruit, or that your depression starts after your vodka. Other people may confuse you, too, by saying vodka stops their depression, or that they never get depression or headaches at all (so therefore you're a hypochondriac).

Our so-called 'normal' diet is a relatively new phenomenon. As Richard Passwater reminds us in *Supernutrition for Healthy Hearts,* we are the first culture ever to derive more than 50 per cent of our calories from processed foods. And Dr Richard Mackarness, the psychiatrist author of *Not All in the Mind — The Hazards of Hidden Allergies,* has this to say:

> Meat has been man's main food for over nine-tenths of his time since he learned to walk upright and use his hands as tools . . . starches and sugars as a basis for nutrition are a very recent introduction; they have been part of our diet for 10 000 years at most, as against 2 or 3 million years on fat, meat and protein.

Put like this, you can see that 10 000 years is just the blink of an eyelid, and the ratio of grain-eating to meat, vegetables, nuts and fruit is around 1:300. In other words, human beings have been eating starches and sugars for a mere 500 generations.

Dr Mackarness writes:

> Our modern carbohydrate-based diet of highly refined and processed foods, contaminated by hundreds of newly invented synthetic chemicals, is such a recent innovation that there has not yet been time for extensive study of its effects on humans.

Most of the evidence beginning to come in, however, suggests that the effects may be harmful.

So, the human race had barely begun to down its daily bread, and old-fashioned wholegrain bread at that, because refining processes weren't commonly used until the 1880s, when it had to adjust to a whole new set of hazardous additives as well.

Sugar? We used to eat only a few pounds per year in the last century. Today, in America, it's one teaspoonful per hour per person throughout life. Which means that for every person who never touches sugar, there's another who's taking two teaspoons per hour, or more. This includes all the hidden sugar added to bread, soups, tinned fruits, soft drinks and cough mixtures.

NUTRITIONAL MEDICINE
The dawn of modern nutritional medicine coincided with the discovery of vitamins and their association with their use in the prevention of diseases. Soon after, however, medical scientists lost interest in these substances because they did not appear to be particularly valuable as a tool against the prevailing illnesses of the times. Medicine became increasingly preoccupied with specific agents (drugs) that were demonstrably able to abate symptoms and cure disease. Little thought was given to the possibility of side-effects or long-term problems thus engendered. Focussing on bacteria, scientists forgot that an invading oganism must enter a weakened, receptive host in order to take up residence and that if the individual's resistance is good, bacteria, viruses and toxic organisms may well remain harmless.

The role played by good nutrition, environment and trace nutrients in maintaining our resistance was not well appreciated. Yet the health of each of our body cells is largely dependent on its environment. What we give them is what they get. Pile in the junk food, take drugs and wash them down with chemicalised water and your liver cells can't just get up and move house. They are stuck! And they begin to suffer. And as a consequence they become less efficient and more prone to bad health.

If this happens to some of the cells of your digestive system, you will suffer poor digestion. If it happens to cells in your ligaments you may have a bad back. Allow your brain cells to live in a toxic or unsuitable environment and your behaviour, moods and emotions will suffer. But just like a suitable environment for a Sydneysider is Sydney, an Eskimo may find that beautiful city far too polluted, hot and generally unsuitable for optimal functioning.

So it is for cells. Some thrive in an extremely acidic environment, others can only function in alkalinity. Some like it hot, some prefer it cold. The requirements of human cells can vary as much as the humans themselves. Logically, the environment for cells can be improved upon and conditions altered in some situations to optimise functions. One of the ways to achieve this is with good nutrition.

We need, at least, some forty odd nutrients. If we eat anything, be it fried camel's feet or steak and eggs or just apples, we get SOME of the nutrients. 'Some', however, may not be enough all the time. And 'some' can be positively bad if we are in an unusual situation — like SICK!

So what will make us better? The answer to that requires a knowledge of the individual far more than knowing what the illness is.

This is where the nutritionist comes in. He/she will investigate you, the individual, taking into account any health problems you have and symptoms you are experiencing, and will come up with a diet for YOU.

FINDING A GOOD NUTRITIONIST

So what can YOU do to make sure you receive the correct nutritional advice? Let me assure you that there are some areas you can, and should explore, alone or together with your therapist, which will help you establish your own biochemical identity.

The first one has a rather frightening title: *anthropometric data*. In plain English this refers to all the data concerning: the health history of your family as well as your own health history; a list of the medications, natural or otherwise, which you have taken, or are currently taking, together with any effects, positive or negative that they may have had on you and on the course of the condition for which they were taken; basic lifestyle habits, such as alcohol consumption, exercise, etc.; the state of your heart, lungs; the results of any previous tests, whether orthodox blood pathology or 'alternative', such as iris diagnosis. Usually a well-designed questionnaire can go a long way in helping a therapist gather relevant information and I would caution a prospective patient to be very wary of any nutritionist that did not use one.

Biochemical data is also very important. Your blood tests results may well have been 'within normal limits' but the experienced therapist will be able to re-interpret them in the light of your biochemical individuality and be on the lookout for *clusters* of low or high parameters, which can point to areas of concern.

Foods for Moods

The brain, like all organs of the body, is made up of individual cells, and each of these cells, again like all those of the body, is made up from the various constituents of the foods you eat and subsequently absorb. Each cell in turn is bathed in a fluid (the cell environment) made up, once more, of what you have ingested — in this case, fluids, minerals, vitamins, glucose, etc. So it is only by eating, breathing or drinking that you can supply your brain cells with their environment.

The brain is composed of around 80 per cent water. Each cell of the brain communicates with others via liquid spaces containing floating chemicals which transmit signals from one brain cell to another with lightning speed. These chemicals are called *neurotransmitters*.

Placing foreign chemicals in the fluid surrounding the brain cells will affect the functioning of the brain as a whole. Alcohol, LSD and amphetamines will all cause changes in the individual whose brain has been exposed to them. But we know that already. What many people don't realise is that even breathing petrol fumes containing lead can alter the composition of these fluids, so that subtle (and eventually not-so-subtle) behaviour changes can occur. Even simple, ordinary, helpful and healthy proteins like gluten may cause some predisposed or hypersensitive brains to react.

Until recently, medical scientists viewed with suspicion claims that ordinary foods and nutrients could affect the brain directly. All of this has changed now. Dr Richard Wurtman, Director of Massachusetts Institute of Technology's Neuroendocrinal Research Laboratory, says:

> Recent experiments at the MIT have demonstrated that certain foods can raise the levels of brain neurotransmitters. Almost all these are made by nerve cells from simple amino acids derived directly from the food one eats, with the help of several vitamin- and mineral-dependent enzymes.

Take a basic function such as memory. Around 1 per cent of the population suffers from a brain deterioration associated with senility, which causes the afflicted to lose his/her memory. Alzheimer's disease, as it is called, strikes around 2 million people each year in the United States. Researchers suspect that an insufficient supply of nutrients is able to reach the brains of these people, and that these same brains are deficient in acetylcholine (ACH), a neurotransmitter. ACH is necessary for cellular communication which, in turn, is partly responsible for what we call 'memory'.

The interesting thing is that the brain makes acetylcholine from choline, a constituent of lecithin, eggs, liver and soya beans, among other foods. Dr Peter Davies, of the British Medical Research Council, has found a positive correlation between Alzheimer's disease and a brain deficiency of acetylcholine. Dr Katherine Bick of NIH has studied the effects of choline supplementation (primarily lecithin) on memory. One study showed enhanced memory and diminished signs of mental confusion among a good portion of the patients. However in some susceptible people, excessive choline may aggravate or even precipitate symptoms of depression. Choline-rich foods may also make you sleepy — ideal if you suffer from insomnia, but not so good if you need to stay alert or are already lethargic.

The power of food to influence human moods may be much greater than we thought. According to Dr G. Schwartz, in his book *Food Power,* it is possible to induce almost any desired state by carefully choosing the type and quantity of food one eats.

Are you overweight? Tired? Lethargic? Always sleepy? Then

avoid foods with poppy seed, cabbage, broccoli, soya beans or peas. They all contain thyroid-inhibiting substances that can aggravate these conditions. At the same time, oysters, shellfish and fish in general are high in iodine and contain some steroids likely to increase your metabolic rate.

Ready to go out for a big night? To paint the town red? Want to increase your libido? Not so difficult with the right menu to help you. First of all, avoid large quantities of carrots, food containing monosodium glutamate, eggs, milk, turkey or pineapple — they all contain tryptophan, which may make you sleepy.

Basil contains a relaxant called methylchavicol, and the humble lettuce at least two substances, lactucin and hyoscyamine, that may relax you too much. Do not eat a lot of watermelon, either. The cucurbocitin in it is very good for lowering the blood pressure, but may make it difficult for you to stay the distance.

Drink up, by all means, but not valerian tea, which contains (among other relaxants) chantinine or anisette (full of methylchavicol), which could also put you 'out' before time. On the other hand, if you make yourself a healthy drink containing spearmint, ginger ale and a dash of cinnamon you have three stimulants going for you — menthol, gingerol and cinnamaldehyde.

Chicken livers, soy sauce, pickled herrings, yoghurt, sour cream, avocados and licorice are all relatively high in tyramine (a stimulant). If you want to do a really good job, try some myrystin (saffron, pepper and nutmeg). Some chocolate, ginseng and vanilla may help, but garlic is sure to do wonders for you. It contains a mild stimulant, but also will make it possible for you to absorb all the vitamin B1 from your food.

The sinigrin in horseradish and borneol in rosemary will enhance the stimulatory effect of chicken, and if you finish off with a good-sized drink of sarsaparilla, you have at least increased the odds in your favour. Very ripe bananas and avocados would make the ideal dessert in this case, as their tyramine content may just be what you need to guarantee a successful evening! If hard spirits are what you like, probably the safest stimulant drink is tequila. It is made from the cactus plant, is non-allergenic, and seems to stimulate more effectively than most liquors.

If you get hungry on the way home, don't stop at a takeaway shop for some chips. Apart from the fact that oils heated to high temperatures, or for a prolonged period of time, are known to be carcinogenic, chips are often made with potatoes that have been bathed in difluorodichloromethane. If this sounds ghastly, it's because *it is ghastly,* especially if it is allowed to react with commonly used pesticides or spray propellants.

PSYCHODIETETICS
This is the study of how foods, chemicals or metals to which one is allergic, hypersensitive or maladapted, can cause mental processes to become unbalanced, thereby producing antisocial, criminal behaviour or psychiatric illnesses.

If you suffer from psychotic depression, poor concentration, hyperactivity, or display criminal tendencies or symptoms of early schizophrenia, it may be that a simple food allergy is the base cause. Today, medical scientists in this field, psychodietetics, are beginning to realise the extent of symptoms and possible causes, and how they relate to well-known patterns of antisocial behaviour.

An increasing number of scientists are becoming convinced that food allergies and other types of hypersensitivities to environmental factors can trigger behaviour which leads to personality problems ranging from depression to psychosis.

Stress

What is stress, exactly? Even the man who invented the stress concept admits it's hard to explain. He's Dr Hans Selye, Professor and Director of the Institute of Experimental Medicine and Surgery at the University of Montreal, in Canada, who holds doctorates in medicine, science and philosophy.

Here's how Dr Selye sees stress:

> Everybody knows what stress is and nobody knows what it is. The word stress, like success, failure or happiness, means different things to different people and, except for a few specialised scientists, no one has really tried to define it, although it has become part of our daily vocabulary. Is it

effort, fatigue, pain, fear, the need for concentration, the humiliation of censure, loss of blood, or even an unexpected success that requires complete reformulation of one's life?

The answer is yes and no. That is what makes the definition of stress so difficult. Every one of these conditions can produce stress, and yet none of them can be singled out as being 'it' since the word applies equally to all others as well.

Tricky, you see? But meanwhile there's one thing we're all sure of. There's more stress about these days. In answer to those old folk who're convinced they had their share of stress in the old days, medical authorities generally point out that in the past it was easier to take some action and 'get it out of your system'.

Our ancestors killed wild animals, ran away from them, or were eaten by them. If they felt cranky, they chopped a load of wood, or perhaps got together with their friends and took the law into their own hands. Even today, there are therapy groups where you're encouraged to whack pillows, and the ancient Chinese idea of a 'screaming room' has its counterpart in many psychiatric hospitals today. When things get too much, you just go in there and give vent to your feelings.

While all this is true to a point, one of our modern ideas about stress isn't true. Somehow, we've got the idea that stress is a terribly bad thing; that if only we could abolish stress people wouldn't have heart attacks and nervous breakdowns. But, as Dr Selye says, we wouldn't have many thrills either, because success, and triumph, may count as stressful, too.

In the words of Dr Selye stress is 'the non-specific response of the body to any demand made upon it'. Note that word, 'non-specific'. Specific responses, that is, the ones you can see, vary. Crying, fainting, shivering, sweating and vomiting are all specific responses; and quite different situations may evoke very similar specific responses. You can laugh till you cry, too, or shiver with pleasant anticipation just as much as from fear.

Non-specific responses are what's going on backstage, so to speak: in order to make all these specific responses possible and then to get the body back to normal after the crisis.

What are these non-specific responses? To understand what's going on in there, it helps to know something about the endocrine system — that part of the body which so often defies conscious control and which taunts us by producing either too many hormones or too few.

The endocrine gland, which gets most of the headlines, is actually a pair — the adrenals — which sit on top of each kidney and behave in a very macho way. Aggression, drive, energy, that's what we associate with the adrenals. But it's not so simple. The adrenal glands consist of two parts — an outer, tough, exterior called the cortex, and a mushier interior called the medulla. Curiously, you may think, it's the soft-centred medulla which produces the adrenalin.

The adrenal medulla, however, and the adrenal cortex, are not the liberated self-starters you might think they are. Both are under the thumb of the pituitary gland, which sits at the base of the brain in a bony hollow known as the 'Turkish saddle', and is about the size of a pea.

The pituitary gland was long considered 'the conductor of the endocrine orchestra'. But it's now known that the pituitary is only a front, too, as it were, and the real godfather of the endocrine organisation seems to be the hypothalamus. This is a tiny pocket, or ventricle, in the brain which acts like a bugging device on all incoming messages about sight, sound, taste, smell. Nothing escapes the attention of the hypothalamus.

With the discovery of the hypothalamus, the old puzzle of how 'nerves' affected body function was solved. The hypothalamus not only has nerves coming in with messages — I'm too hot/cold, I can smell apple pie/aftershave/something burning — but translates these nerve messages into chemical substances called releasing factors. These travel down the little stalk connecting it to the pituitary and set its hormones off.

The adrenal medulla, the soft inner core, is all about nerve messages, too — from the autonomic, or involuntary, nervous system. And when alarm bells sound, whether they're actual ones or silent cries for help from an enzyme in distress, adrenalin pours into the bloodstream to make the heart pump faster, to narrow the blood vessels so that pressure will rise and send the oxygen where it's needed. The lungs and air passages relax, too, to help the oxygen supply still further. Blood tends to be drawn toward the muscles, in readiness for action, leaving the face white and the digestion interrupted (there are more important things to do now, the body thinks).

That's not the end of the story. When the adrenalin reaches the pituitary, it begins to secrete chemicals, or hormones, which zoom down via the bloodstream to the adrenal cortex which has thirty-two of its own chemicals/hormones ready to spring into action. Meanwhile, the thyroid, the parathyroid, the sex glands and a portion of the pancreas get the green light, too, to secrete their particular hormones.

The end result of all this chemical sleight-of-hand, which happens just about as quickly as any stage magician's trick, is sometimes a superhuman feat of strength and quick-wittedness, such as we know people can perform in dire emergencies. Frail women lift fallen trees off trapped children, athletes or VC winners perform incredible feats of endurance that surprise even themselves, afterwards.

But it's when strength, speed, and quick-wittedness are not going to solve the problem that it can get serious. For instance, it is inappropriate to punch your boss or the policeman who has pulled you over.

As you can see, the result of the adrenal alarm going off is to send little shock waves into just about every corner of your body, revving it up, as it were, for action. A major group of substances released by the adrenal cortex is the glucocorticoids, which obligingly shoot up the blood-sugar level so you'll have more energy, relying on the trusty pancreas to secrete the insulin to bring the sugar level down when the excitement's over.

So even a candy bar can act as a form of stress. Not only does the pancreas resent having to rush out and deal with the extra blood sugar if it happens too often, but it may overreact so violently that more blood sugar has to be created at all costs. To satisfy this the body starts dipping into its capital reserves.

More bad news. The adrenal cortex also secretes cortisone, which damps down the body's immune responses. You don't want to be worried about a scratch or two in a crisis, do you? And we've all heard of sportsmen, or soldiers, not only peforming amazing physical feats but performing them despite quite serious injuries. Broken toes, broken ribs, in the heat of the moment they simply don't notice.

This may be a good thing, short-term, but if the body's immune responses get the feeling nobody wants them, then some major actors assume they're superfluous and retire in a huff —

the lymph nodes. The purpose of the lymph nodes is to fight infections. In cases of organ transplants, when it's clearly better if the body doesn't get alarmed about strange tissues taking up residence, a slumbering lymph system is of great benefit. But otherwise, no.

The thymus gland does most of its work before birth and in early childhood, teaching little antibodies the difference between friend and foe so that the body won't start attacking itself, as sometimes happens in autoimmune diseases. The thymus begins to dwindle after puberty; but there's impressive evidence that the thymus is something of a biological regulator; the longer it functions the greater the lifespan.

Then there's the thyroid gland, which gets the message from the pituitary to turn up the body's thermostat, that is, to increase metabolism. This means fat stores are raided to make extra energy, body protein may be broken down, and calcium is seconded from the bones — a situation very like the scene in *Go West* where the Marx Brothers chop up the train for fuel. Vitamins are used up more quickly; the gastrointestinal tract races overtime, sometimes to the point of producing diarrhoea. And obviously no thyroid gland is going to work overtime too long before complaining.

It's when the emergency doesn't end, and you're still huffing and fuming six hours later with no solution in sight, that the situation can get serious.

Putting all these assorted miseries and malfunctions of the endocrine system together into a neat 'stress concept of disease' was what Dr Selye eventually did. What follows is a summary of his conclusions.

In the face of continuing stress the body goes through three phases. Firstly, alarm bells ring and the body reacts directly to the stress. Then comes adaptation to the situation and increased resistance. The final phase is exhaustion and collapse.

In the second stage of adaptation, or resistance, the behaviour of the body is quite different, even the exact opposite, to what it was in the alarm situation. And the shrunken thymus glands and enlarged adrenal cortexes and bleeding ulcers — all signs of stage two — reminded Dr Selye that he'd seen much the same thing in sick people, not just in rats. Privately, he'd always referred to these non-specific signs as 'the syndrome of just being sick', and he'd found it puzzling that they occurred in all kinds of patients, whether they had an infectious disease or cancer.

Dr Selye began to think that illnesses might not be caused directly by any one particular germ, or virus, but by faulty adaptive responses to the stress caused by these things: for instance, various emotional disturbances, headaches, insomnia, upset stomachs, sinus, hypertension, gastric and duodenal ulcers, some types of rheumatism and allergies, and cardiovascular and kidney diseases.

Over the years, other doctors had noticed much the same thing as Hans Selye had: the enlarged, bloodshot, adrenal glands of guinea pigs with diphtheria, the ulcers in people who'd suffered extensive skin burns. But somehow they'd never followed it through and nailed stress as the culprit.

WHY DOES STRESS AFFECT DIFFERENT PEOPLE DIFFERENTLY?

We all know that tension around the office, or at the breakfast table, can give one person hypertension, another one ulcers, and yet another a headache or a pain in the neck.

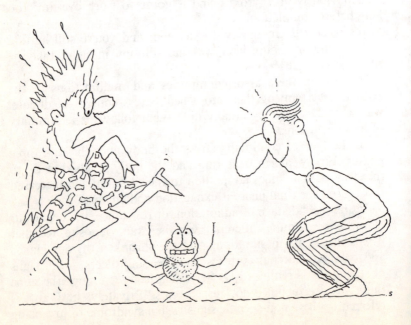

Dr Selye figured out that this was because people are individuals and laboratory rats aren't. Animals used in experiments tend to be the same breed, the same age, and perhaps even from the same litter — which in human terms means it's like asking all 40-year-old American women if they were ever in love with Elvis Presley. Picked out at random in the streets of New York human beings are not like peas in a pod. They have environmental differences, hereditary weaknesses, different occupational stresses and different emotional reactions to similar events. It's all a question of where the weak link is.

HOW TO DEAL WITH STRESS

The burning question as far as you're concerned, seeing stress is a part of life whether you're rich, poor, male, female, old, young, black or white, is how to deal with it.

With a little practice and determination, you may learn to enjoy some of your stresses, to welcome them as wonderful challenges and the spice of life. It's hard to teach an old dog new tricks, but sometimes an expert therapist can help.

Try to establish what it is you really want from life and, if you're not happy, stop doing what other people think you ought to be doing. Try to be a graceful loser, and to develop the knack of knowing when a thing's worth getting steamed up about and when it isn't. Hans Selye uses the illustration of an innocent bystander menaced by a belligerent drunk: clearly the most sensible thing is to ignore him and walk by. As Alcoholics Anonymous might say in their Serenity Prayer: 'God grant me the serenity to accept the things I cannot change, courage to change the things I can, and wisdom to know the difference'.

Dr Selye's most important piece of advice is exactly what this book is about. Nobody knows your stress thresholds better than you do, he says; so try being your own doctor. You should be able to feel instinctively when you've had enough, when it's time to switch off, to quit. Each individual must find his/her own level of stress, because below that you'll feel bored and frustrated, and above that you'll suffer exhaustion.

Reactions to stress may vary, but research shows that a tremendous number of unexplainable illnesses occur within a short time after an individual has been exposed to a particular major stressor.

There is also strong evidence that different personality types are more prone to their own kind of disease, whether it is heart attack, cancer, arthritis, stomach ulcers, rheumatoid arthritis, asthma or urinary infections. There is a growing body of opinion that this is because it is how the different personality types handle stress that is the key to their illnesses. Chinese medicine and acupuncture have known this for centuries. Bear in mind that apart from the effect of personality, biochemical individuality also plays a part. Genetically, everyone's system is different and the 'weak link in the chain' varies accordingly.

All forms of stress can cause degenerative disease in the long run because of the non-specific responses they provoke in the body. And now, at last, we are beginning to understand how hypersensitivity to food, and to chemicals and pollutants in our environment, can work together to act as yet another stress.

While there is not a clear-cut cause-and-effect situation — that is, 'If you eat such and such you will definitely get this disease' — you will, over a period of time, find that exposure to chemicals, plus the stresses of modern life, plus the stresses of the animals and birds whose bodies we eat, plus the maladaptive reaction to the relatively new foods in our diet like wheat, corn and milk, may add up to bodily disease. Any one of these factors may be the last straw which breaks the camel's (your) back.

REDUCING STRESS
While there's nothing this book can do to prevent external stresses — because we can't exchange your husband or your child or your boss — we can make sure that you're not adding to the turmoil that's going on inside your body by taking on extra stresses.

Since one of the royal roads by which stress can get a hold on the body is via the mouth, you can, first of all, find out (and this book will show you how) whether you're not well adapted to a certain type of diet: for instance, whether vegetarianism is really for you.

Then, if we can find what general type of diet suits you, we can be more specific. What vegetables are for you? Which grains should you eat, or avoid? And, therefore, which types of alcohol?

The third step is to avoid any chemicals that are added, perhaps with the best of intentions, to your food. You can't stop breathing, but you can get a filter for your drinking water, and you can try to buy food that is unadulterated. You can try to eat more fresh food, and so on.

Because the body's ability to stand up to this sort of stress is indirectly dependent on the proper complement of vitamins and minerals to help your enzymes function properly, an adequate supply of these, plus specific vitamins to suit your individual needs, will also help your body's resistance to stress.

By following these steps, you can eliminate those stresses in your life that are avoidable. You've avoided smoking? Good, because that's a major stress. So is alcohol, and so is working fourteen hours a day. But if you have to work fourteen hours a day, and like a certain amount of alcohol, don't despair, because you can still even things up. For instance, by eating less white sugar and more fresh vegetables.

Already there are people who seem to understand this credit-debit approach to health. It's not uncommon today to find smokers who take more care of their diet than do non-smokers, or people who'll eat dessert only if they've faithfully stuck to their exercise schedule. They're not fooling themselves either. Because little things do make a difference, and these people have grasped an essential point — that health is about balance.

You do not necessarily have the same capacity for withstanding life's trials as your friends. Your drinking, smoking, even overweight or hysterical, friends, may just happen to have unusually high thresholds, that is, good resistance. While virtuous little you may be knocked out by the lowest rating stresses of all — minor violations of the law, like getting a parking ticket. If you have no reserves, no money in the bank for a stress emergency, it's not a minor stress at all.

CFS — An Overview

Just What is CFS?

Chronic Fatigue Syndrome (CFS) is a hard illness to classify. The fact that it is not a disease, but a syndrome makes it even harder. And for this reason, despite medical literature going back some fifty years, many doctors still consider CFS as 'all in the mind' of the sufferer. In 1986, Dr Victor Herbert, a very influential physician in the United States, described CFS as an 'imaginary disease' and suggested that sufferers should be treated as psychiatric cases and given medications and treatments suitable for such patients.

On the other hand, Dr Anthony Kormakoff, head of a Harvard medical school teaching hospital and a leading United States CFS researcher, is convinced that the illness is real.

In 1987 he said:

> The symptoms [of CFS] are clearly organic, and many quite severe. Differentiation is difficult, except in degree, between myalgic encephalomyelitis, the chronic viral fatigue syndrome, 'true' chronic mononucleosis [Epstein Barr-induced chronic glandular fever], severe chronic active EBV infections, and fibrositis.

In 1983 a major outbreak of what we now know was CFS occurred in New Zealand, in a little town by the name of Tapanui. It appeared to be triggered off by an 'Asian' flu epidemic which involved the Coxakie B virus. The outbreak was given the name 'Tapanui Flu' and that only served to confuse the matter further. Whole families were stricken and around 15 per cent of the population was affected. Coincidentally, Tapanui is in the middle of a rural area which also has one of the world's highest incidences of cot deaths, multiple sclerosis, arthritis and asthma.

Jay Goldstein, a psychoneuroimmunologist (a scientist who studies the link between the mind, disease and immunity) at the University of California, says of CFS:

> To me, this is the most complex disease of all modern medicine because there are so many variables. It makes people wonder if the way it works is beyond the capacity of the human brain to understand.

Perhaps one of the problems is the fact that people in the 1990s are really a new breed. We are different biochemically and genetically from humans of the 1950s. Perhaps antibiotics, insulin, the pill and countless other drugs, plus the myriad of chemicals we litter our environment with, have changed the genetic and physiological make-up of some of the people more frequently exposed to them. Such changes may be very subtle. Too subtle for our methods of measurement, until they trigger something off.

Orthodox medical textbooks and much of medical training may well be geared to diagnose and treat people who no longer exist.

The CFS Puzzle

There are many and very complex reasons why it has taken such a long time for CFS to be recognised, and even more reasons for the failure of so many medical, and even some alternative medicine's, practitioners to understand this syndrome, its many causes and manifestations, and the consequences for their patients' health.

Among these reasons is the fact that scientific discoveries and findings can take a long time, even years, to reach the medical literature. Even then, they may be first published in some obscure journal long before they make their way slowly to the more generally read publications. In some instances, new findings may lie buried in a report for a long time for unusual reasons. For example, it has been known since the early 1980s that drinking a moderate amount of alcohol with your meals actually protects people against heart disease, and that mortality rates from all causes are lower for moderate drinkers than for teetotallers and heavy drinkers (the so-called U effect). A couple of glasses of wine with your meals not only tends to lower total cholesterol but it also lowers the more dangerous type of cholesterol (LDL), while enhancing that of the protective cholesterol (HDL).

In fact, it has been stated that this measure will lower cholesterol and reduce the chances of heart disease more and better than any dietary changes.

Yet these findings were not made public, even to many doctors, until early 1991, partly because authorities feared it may encourage drinking and add to the already enormous alcohol-abuse problems in our society.

Many, if not all the factors involved in CFS have been studied and reported for many years in the literature. Indeed, CFS is not new at all; but pieces of the puzzle are still only emerging.

SOME PIECES OF THE PUZZLE

It is clear that CFS can be caused by a latent virus. In fact, the symptoms of the so-called Post Viral Syndrome or Chronic Epstein Barr Virus Syndrome (CEBVS) are indistinguishable from CFS. It is also quite obvious that viruses will produce such effects only in susceptible individuals and history has shown that the number of such individuals is climbing steadily.

We also know that CFS can be caused by the influence of chemicals, by immuno-incompetence, mitochondrial damage, even electromagnetic radiation. Or it can be caused by any of the myriad possible interactions of these factors.

But, irrespective of its cause, CFS tends to disrupt our defence mechanisms.

In our experience we have learnt that so many of the symptoms of CFS, such as chronic candida infections, intestinal/digestive problems (malabsorption, dysbiosis, parasitic infections, intestinal thrush, food allergies, etc.) and environmental allergies/hypersensitivities, to name but a few, can cause illnesses with symptoms similar and often identical to those of CFS or can affect our immune system so that we are more likely to become victims of CFS.

Viruses
As I already pointed out, the symptoms of a patient suffering

the effects of the Post Viral Fatigue Syndrome or one with Chronic Epstein Barr Virus Syndrome (CEBVS) will be very difficult, if not impossible, to distinguish from those of CFS.

But, in spite of the fact that innumerable clues appeared in many scientific journals, it was not until August 1989 that the general scientific literature published the first official proof. In that month, *Scientific American* carried an article (later appearing also in the *New England Journal of Medicine*) by Professor Michael Oldstone, an immunologist and neuropharmacologist working at the Scripp Clinic and Research Foundation in La Jolla, California, entitled 'Viral Alteration of Cell Functions'.

The article described quite clearly how it is quite possible for a virus to enter a body and take up permanent residence without provoking any of the symptoms usually associated with a viral infection, other than perhaps a transient, mild flu-like feeling.

Professor Oldstone also plainly demonstrated that such viruses can then act insidiously to alter cell functions, neurotransmitters, hormone production and secretion, enzyme production, immune responses and even myocardial (heart muscle) contractions in such ways that they may be responsible for such varied diseases as growth retardation, diabetes, neuropsychiatric disorders (depression, anxiety, emotional liability, nervous tension, mental illness, etc.), autoimmune disease (lupus, SLE, arthritis, multiple sclerosis, etc.), blood sugar metabolism aberrations and even heart disease. The author suggests that many other illnesses, not previously thought to have a viral infectious cause, may thus be indirectly caused by viruses.

We already know that viruses affect our immune system. What the good professor demonstrated was the ability of these agents to prevent the formation of some of the B cells and to interfere with the ability of some of the T cells known as cytotoxic T8, to destroy infected cells. They discovered, in other words, that persistent viral infection, even in the absence of symptoms, can alter the physiological functions of cells without destroying them. This is achieved by interfering with cells called T8 so that the number of these cells circulating is not reduced — just their competence. Meanwhile the host cell's own life-sustaining functions are left alone and provide the virus with a comfortable home, full of the substances it needs to survive and multiply.

Put simply, this means that the viruses do not kill outright some of the 'soldiers' that make up our defences; they just render them less efficient at doing their job, that is, fighting for our good health. Unfortunately there is a tendency among medical scientists to behave like sheep farmers: to count them as they go through the gate rather than try to ascertain the health of each individual sheep, or cell.

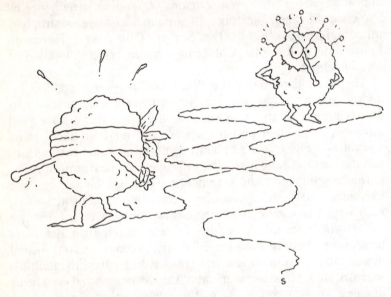

The paper also describes how viruses can affect the production of hormones and, indirectly, almost any gland in the body, from the thyroid to the adrenal.

Professor Oldstone simply confirms what so many of us have believed for some time. That post viral syndromes can and do cause chronic fatigue and that what has been known as the Chronic Epstein Barr Virus Syndrome or Sub-Clinical Immune Dysregulation Syndrome (SCIDS) can often be CFS and vice versa.

Candida
The next missing piece of the CFS puzzle concerns a yeast fungus (a form of mould) called *Candida albicans*. In 1987, Drs Jonathon Brostoff, Honorary Consultant Physician at the Department of Immunology at Middlesex Hospital and Medical School in

London (UK) and Stephen Challacombe, Honorary Consultant at the Department of Oral Immunology and Microbiology at the United Medical and Dental Schools of Guy's and St Thomas Hospitals, London (UK), published a book entitled *Food Allergies*.

In a chapter of this book, which detailed the symptoms of a syndrome known as Autoimmune, Polyendocrinopathy, Immune Dysregulation, Candidiasis, Hypersensitivity Syndrome (APICH), they described quite clearly how *Candida albicans* can cause allergies, infect people and disrupt their immune systems. It can cause the body to start making antibodies against several organs/systems and precipitate, aggravate and even initiate many a disease. (Sound familiar?) Then, in 1989 Professor Cora Saltarelli, a research scientist renowned for her invention of a new method for separating and scanning organic cells and molecules, wrote a book entitled *Candida albicans — The Pathogenic Fungus* in which she describes, documents and explains in no uncertain terms how *Candida albicans* can affect the human immune system as well as contribute to a considerable number of illnesses ranging from heart disease to kidney problems.

This is one of the reasons why you will find a whole chapter of my book devoted to candida.

As you are aware by now, many people suffering with CFS are also affected by candida. You may also know that candida sufferers, as well as CFS sufferers, are emotionally labile. In other words, they tend to be anxious, tense, moody, teary, aggressive, depressed and/or generally a little bit neurotic.

We have been noting for a long time that people who suffer with chronic candida infections, post viral syndromes, hypoglycaemia and CFS, tend to be emotionally unstable. We know this is so in many people affected by latent viruses. In 1977 I observed the same mood problems in a group of depressed female patients who did not respond to either conventional or nutritional/ orthomolecular treatment. After a time I realised that they were suffering from chronic candida infections and, after treating this condition, I found that all their 'mental' symptoms disappeared.

More recently we have learned that fungi (the word 'fungi' is synonymous with 'mould') can produce powerful toxins and that these can provoke a disastrous array of symptoms in some patients. The *New Scientist* article describes in great detail how common fungi can produce a special type of poison known as *gliotoxin,* which attacks a particular group of brain cells. These gliotoxins can kill cells and severely damage the immune system. So much so they are being considered as useful but 'natural' drugs to combat cancer and safeguard organ transplants against rejection by the host's immune system.

In fact, already one of the most commonly used drugs by surgeons to stop organs rejection is Cyclosporin A. It is actually made by the fungus *Tolypocladium gams.* Other moulds are also capable of influencing our immune system, notably *Aspergillus fumigatus* and *Penicillium notatum.*

If only medical doctors were forced to read the scientific literature and keep up to date! When a patient with a well-established allergy to moulds, who lives in a home full of fungi, eats foods containing mould, breathes air laden with mould spores and suffers with recurrent candida infections, dares to imply that these factors may contribute to his/her mood swings, some general practitioners dismiss the whole thing as a figment of the patient's aberrant imagination and often label him/her 'neurotic'.

Xenobiotics
The next piece of the CFS puzzle should not even be missing because it has been so obvious for the past twenty years. It concerns xenobiotics (foreign chemicals).

For the life of me, I cannot understand how anyone can fail to appreciate that adding many thousands of NEW toxic chemicals to our environment for years on end (at least for the past forty years) is going to affect the health of human beings. Especially since these chemicals are used to kill animal cells, to strip protective coatings from enzymes, to use up precious, and often scarce, reserves of essential minerals, enzymes, vitamins and amino acids.

Yet even this simple fact failed to make an impact on grass-root practitioners because, just like in the case of viruses, people were not aware that a crucial and extremely fragile part of our cells called the mitochondria (also known as the 'powerhouses of the cells') can be damaged by a variety of factors, including chemicals, and that this can give rise to serious illnesses (even a few that we thought were hereditary) in some individuals while leaving others unscathed. Then, in mid-1989, Anthony Ninnane, an Australian molecular biologist at Monash University in Victoria (Australia), showed that mitochondrial damage may be actually responsible for cellular ageing. Because the mitochondria are essential for providing energy to cells, and therefore to every system in the body, a reduction in the functions of some of their enzymes leads to an impairment of cellular respiration.

Cells, like us, cannot perform efficiently without a form of 'breathing' and when this is damaged they wind down. Groups of tissues follow and eventually organs or systems join the list. Eventually the whole body simply winds down, we age, become ill and eventually die. Ninnane is now considering the use of vitamin C and other antioxidant substances in the hope of replenishing or repairing the depleted/damaged mitochondrial enzymes.

We have known about and studied the ageing process since science began. And we know only too well that ageing and disease often go hand in hand. Controversial as the subject may be, almost all researchers in the field agree on one point. Oxidation produces 'free radicals' and free radicals are involved in cellular ageing, disease states and death.

Every chemical added to our environment tends to increase the amount of free radicals generated and decrease the body's ability to detoxify. We all know some of these chemicals are bad because they may cause cancer or affect foetuses. What some people do not realise is that, in far more subtle ways, they may contribute to an acceleration of the ageing process and the promotion of a variety of degenerative diseases by slowly impairing our immune system. Viral diseases, candida and a host of other illnesses are caused by OPPORTUNISTIC organisms and only occur when our resistance is compromised. Even low-grade, chronic exposure to chemicals can render one more susceptible to allergies, biochemical aberrations and immune disorders such as arthritis.

How do xenobiotics affect us?

Whenever the molecular basis for ageing and illness is discussed, there is little doubt in the mind of most research scientists that it is the effect of *free radicals*. Technically, a free radical is a reactive molecule with one electron missing.

The process called metabolism is essential to life. It consists of eating and drinking, digesting, extracting nutrients and energy from the foods and producing heat as a result of this. Imagine living in a big empty room on a very cold, snowbound mountaintop. Imagine a nice fireplace with a wood fire going full blast. You need this to keep warm; you need it to survive. The bigger the fire, the greater the heat. Our metabolism is just like that fire. It keeps us warm and makes life possible. Indeed, the more you eat and the more you metabolise, as when running for instance, the more heat you generate. Now you know one of the reasons why joggers perspire so copiously. The metabolic process of that fire is called *oxidation*. And oxidation produces free radicals.

In the metabolism-fireplace analogy note that, inevitably, some sparks will fly out of the fire. And land on your carpet. This will damage the carpet. Maybe only a tiny little bit, but damage it, it will. After many, many years of this, the carpet may simply disintegrate.

Well now, the fire is our metabolism. The flying sparks are the inevitable free radicals which are always produced as a result of our metabolic fire; and the carpet is us. Eventually, we all disintegrate and die, largely because of the cumulative effects of innumerable free radical assaults. The bigger the fire, the more sparks, and the sooner one may die, or become ill.

Lymphocytes (an essential part of our resistance — immune system) are highly sensitive to oxidation and free radicals.

If we place a screen in front of the fire, we are going to get much less damage from flying sparks. In addition, if we run around chasing every spark as it lands on the carpet and we step on it very quickly, we minimise any damage the free radicals (sparks) can do. On the other hand, if we fan and fuel the fire further, we are going to provoke more sparks (free radicals).

Most of the toxic chemicals we are exposed to because of pollution are like that. They increase the formation of free radicals. As in the analogy with our fireplace, if we create too many sparks (free radicals) our natural screen may not be enough protection and we may not be able to stop the spread of free radicals. So when you read about chemicals in our air, water, food or beaches, remember that eating, drinking, breathing and even touching them almost invariably adds to the formation of free radicals.

We all have a screen in front of our inner fire (metabolism) which prevents many sparks from landing on our carpet. It is called the *antioxidant metabolism* and it consists of many enzyme systems, like MFO (mixed functions oxidase system), liver factors, amino acids and substances with totally unpronounceable names like glutathione and SODs (super oxide dismutases).

Antioxidants *help* our natural defences (the immune system). Most cells which are capable of eating-up (phagocytic) bacteria and foreign invaders are easily inactivated by oxidants and rely heavily on antioxidants for survival and for their efficiency. And we also have many substances which run around all day like crazy stepping on (it's actually called squelching or scavenging) our metabolic sparks (the free radicals). These substances are known as 'free radical scavengers'.

You may recognise some of them. They are called vitamin E (alpha tocopherol), vitamin A, beta carotene, vitamin C, dimethylglycine (vitamin B15 — also known as pangamic acid), ubiquinone (co-enzyme Q10), zinc, copper, selenium, uric acid, tyrosamine, methionine, cytosine, taurine and several others. Usually the whole group is known as 'the antioxidants'. You can easily see then that if the total free radicals produced by our metabolism via oxidation exceed our defence capabilities (antioxidants) we are in trouble. That is why one of the very few procedures which has been proven to increase lifespan is a reduction in total calories intake. The less calories, the less metabolism, and this means less oxidation and free radicals.

Now let's go back to the sparks (free radicals). We can't stop eating and breathing. But we should minimise any other, non-metabolic, source of oxidation.

So, what are some of the sources of *added* oxidative stress and free radicals? Most, but not all, of them are *xenobiotic* compounds. That rather frightful word means 'foreign compounds not normally found in living systems'. In other, and simpler, words, most human-made chemicals, or, if you prefer, pollutants.

Do I Have CFS?

The onset of CFS can be gradual, developing over months or

even years, or it can be sudden. The pattern can be one of constant malaise with unrelenting symptoms or a spontaneously remitting course with frequent, unexplainable relapses. The symptoms of this disease are quite variable, with new, and sometimes totally unexpected symptoms appearing during the course of the illness. It is not uncommon, for instance, for patients to become suddenly allergic when no allergies were ever experienced before.

SYMPTOMS
Apart from debilitating FATIGUE, the most prominent symptoms appear in the areas of *muscular* and *neuropsychiatric functioning,* although *gastrointestinal-tract (GIT) dysfunctions, multiple allergies* and *infections* are also commonly reported.

Muscular symptoms include general migratory aches and pains as well as exercise-induced muscular fatigue with myalgia (muscular pain and inflammation).
Neuropsychiatric symptoms include difficulties with concentration, memory lapses, emotional lability, mood swings, depression, anxiety, especially LIAS (Lactate Induced Anxiety Syndrome), agoraphobia and, in women, an aggravation of pre-menstrual tension symptoms.
GI symptoms include indigestion, abdominal bloating, constipation or diarrhoea, malabsorption, intestinal thrush and sometimes irritable bowel.
Multiple allergies and infections symptoms include food intolerances, inhalant allergies (dust, dust mites, moulds/fungi, grasses, etc.), sensitivities to common chemicals (pesticides, pollution, car exhaust, etc.), sinusitis, hay fever, asthma, post-nasal drip, excessive throat mucus, skin problems (eczema, dermatitis, etc.).

Many people do not realise that a sudden onset of allergies is a common and well documented result of viral infections (*Annals of Internal Medicine,* 1985) and that when the immune system becomes confused by various attacks it can begin to send out antibodies against everything even vaguely irritating, such as dust, and even against tissues of one's own body (autoimmune disease).

Imagine a terrorist's attack, say a bomb, in the middle of a large city. Chances are the police, tactical response group, army etc. would respond by frantically looking for suspects near the scene of the conflagration. In the course of this search it is quite possible that some people would be investigated, detained and perhaps even arrested, simply because they LOOKED suspicious. A panicky immune system can react just like that — one possible result could be a sudden, new allergy!

Other symptoms. There may be mild elevation of temperature, a fever or a feeling of being cold all the time, joint aches (arthralgia), headaches, lymph node swelling (lymphadenopathy — usually in cases of viral CFS), sore throats and recurrent opportunistic infections such as *Candida albicans*. In addition, sufferers tend to catch frequent colds and flu.

The symptoms can vary from quite mild to severe and even incapacitating. It has been said of CFS that although it will not kill you, it makes some sufferers wish they were dead.

There are many similarities between this cluster of symptoms and that which can occur with APICHS, chronic yeast infections (candida), hypoglycaemia, food intolerances, environmental and inhalant allergies, chemical sensitivities, xenobiotic overload, Epstein Barr, toxoplasmosis, cytomegalovirus, coxackie (or other enteroviruses) and herpes virus type 6 infections.

And on top of all that, the APICH Syndrome and the Chronic Epstein Barr Virus or Post Viral Fatigue Syndromes are often almost indistinguishable from CFS.

WHY YOU MIGHT SUSPECT YOU HAVE CFS

- Suspect CFS if you have seen several doctors, complaining of lots of symptoms which include loss of energy, and still do not have a conclusive diagnosis.
- Consider CFS when the diagnosis that has been made proves to be wrong after further tests.
- The same applies if you know you are quite normal but have been told you are 'neurotic', 'hysterical' or that 'It's all in your head'.
- Note that chemical overload and sensitivity, as well as viral illness, allergies, chronic candida infections and hypoglycaemia, can elicit symptoms which can mimic almost any disease.

- Consider CFS when you have been told that your problem is due to a particular organ dysfunction (liver, digestive system, etc.) without any reason being given for why this should have happened. Also suspect are such vague diagnoses as poor elimination due to bad eating habits, without having been told exactly what the bad habits are and how they could cause the condition.
- Always keep in mind that what are 'good' habits for someone else could turn out to be very bad for you. Every week I see at least one unfortunate person who is allergic to grains (gluten) and became very ill only after switching to a diet very high in complex carbohydrates like bran.
- Suspect something if you live or have lived near a power station, in heavily polluted areas or places known to have been heavily contaminated, or if you work in an industry that uses lots of chemicals, such as agricultural farming, plastics, rubber manufacturing, etc.
- Note if any relatives or people you have had close contact with have had any viral illnesses or if you have had recurrent bouts of flu or other unconfirmed viral attacks which were dismissed as a 'bug that's going around'.
- Consider CFS if, in spite of a good diet and supplements, you suffer with chronic or recurring infections, candida, allergies or such immune diseases as arthritis, lupus, diabetes, multiple sclerosis, cancer, thyroid problems, etc.
- Remember that even if you are found to be chemically sensitive, or overloaded with toxins, and even if positive identification of a viral culprit is made, it is still possible that you suffer other, concurrent health problems with different causes which may need different treatment.
- Make sure you see a diagnostician/therapist who knows how to order and interpret the special tests needed.
- Make sure you and your doctor understand the concept of total load.

DIAGNOSING CFS

It seems logical that to diagnose an illness one needs to know the causes. With syndromes, however, this is not always the case because the cause is usually not known and because any of the presenting symptoms COULD be an illness in its own right and, as in the case of CFS, perhaps be the cause of the major problem.

No wonder then, that when presented with such an evasive entity, everybody (those who don't just simply give up, that is) tries to narrow the symptoms cluster so that an identifiable, underlying cause for the whole bunch can be found!

Yet, time and time again I, and many other diagnosticians, have found that once a cause has been assumed and treatment given SOME of the symptoms persist, although the patient is much better overall, and *could* be defined as being 'cured' of CFS. In such cases it becomes clear that those symptoms have separate causes which have to be found and treated separately. Sometimes we even find that once the cause, say a chemical overload or viral activity, has been ascertained and successfully treated, later events can prove that another 'cause' also exists, and that IT also needs to be treated.

To add to the confusion there is the clinical reality that many practitioners have to face. They treat a patient's symptoms successfully with one method, only to find that when the same method is used to treat the same symptom in another patient with CFS, or when another practitioner tries the same manoeuvre, the result is total failure and, in some cases, even a worsening of the symptom.

As an example, evidence has been presented by some physicians of incredible improvements in energy and stamina after a few weeks of gradually increasing exercise. Others report the opposite. In my own clinical experience, strenuous exercise has always made things worse for the patient.

Then there are other procedures, like saunas, fasting, chelation therapy, ozone infusions, etc., which some find helpful and some find counterproductive. One other glaring example is fasting. If one subjected ALL CFS patients to a fast, one would find the same sort of results one would obtain with any other single procedure. Some would get better, some would get worse, and some would not change.

The reasons are fairly simple. Fasting may mobilise some of the toxic chemicals from the fat of an overweight individual and cause toxic poisoning. Another individual, who is not overweight, may not have the same problem. If the offending chemical is stored in the bones, as lead is, fasting will help, but exercise may kill. If one is very allergic to one or more foods and THAT is slowing down the capacity of the body to fight CFS or slowing down the efficiency of the treatment, then fasting will help a lot. If the immune disturbances are virally induced, fasting may make them very, very much worse and even preclude further improvement for a very long time.

When confronted by patients suffering with CFS day after day, for years on end, as my colleagues and I are, it is sometimes difficult to even start on the road to recovery until the patient gives up his/her negative attitudes. Often, far too often, a patient will declare: 'I have tried EVERYTHING, to no avail. I am not getting any better and I think I may just give up. Obviously there is no hope for me. I'll just have to learn to live with it.'

My colleague Mark Donohoe and I hear this, or something like it, almost every day.

Mark uses a wonderful analogy to make his patients motivated. It goes like this: 'If your boat had three anchors hooked to the sea floor and you pulled two of them up, the boat would still not move an inch. Only when the third one is up will you get going.'

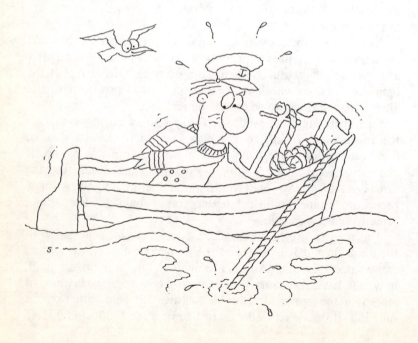

In the case of CFS the rules for diagnosis are controversial, to say the least.

The conventional medicine view
The three medically accepted diagnostic criteria are:

1. Severe, chronic and recurring muscular fatigue, pains, aches or stiffness, that is brought on or aggravated by even slight physical exertion. This condition must have been present for six months or more.
2. Disturbances of the nervous system with mood, emotional or psychiatric disorders, associated with depression, inability to concentrate, short term memory impairment and anxiety.
3. An abnormal cell-mediated immune response, as shown by either a reduction in the number of T cells, an abnormal ratio of some of the T cells or an abnormal response to certain other immunological tests such as the delayed type sensitivity skin test.

The alternative medicine view
Environmental medicine specialists apply a much broader interpretation, as do most alternative medicine practitioners.

In addition, many therapists apply their own individual criteria and may have the tendency to consider some symptoms or a certain cluster of symptoms as being more important than others.

In general, however, they all tend to agree that CFS is either a viral or an environmental syndrome. One must also consider that the many sub-illnesses of CFS can, under some circumstances, be so debilitating that they cause symptoms very similar to those of CFS. For this reason I tend to include these as causes of CFS-like illnesses.

Generally speaking the main diagnostic criteria is that of inexplicable tiredness, with a degree of muscular weakness and mood disturbance, which has not improved after medical (and sometimes alternative) methods of healing.

The syndrome is clinically non-specific and because there is no single test for CFS as such, ANY attempt at a diagnosis must first be one of exclusion. Because of this, the diagnostician first tries to eliminate any serious underlying pathology such as cancer, lupus, Addison's disease, diabetes, etc. During the diagnostic work-up, one has to remember that many CFS symptoms are manifestations of the inter-relationship between the immune and the nervous systems.

DIAGNOSIS
The diagnosis of CFS involves an elimination process.

Muscular symptoms

The muscular symptoms sometimes require a neurological investigation to eliminate the possibility of severe underlying conditions such as MS, motor neuron disease, etc., but generally speaking there is little one can look for in the case of CFS. Gentle massage will sometimes help sufferers, especially in cases of chemical CFS. With viral CFS massage will sometimes aggravate the pains and aches. The problem with inflammation, of any kind, is that tests are only useful when the process reaches a certain stage.

Neuropsychiatric symptoms

The neuropsychiatric symptoms need careful evaluation. We use the HOD (Hoffer & Osmond Diagnostic) test to rule out schizophrenia, suicidal tendencies, paranoia and clinical depression.

Depression is such a common symptom of CFS, yet it can be a clinical entity of its own accord and one has to rule out such types of depression as reactive depression, manic (bi-polar) depression, manic depressive psychosis, SAD (seasonal affective disorder) and depression due to nutritional deficiencies and imbalances. From hypoglycaemia to vitamin B6 deficiencies and from serotonin to norepinephrine abnormalities — the possibilities are numerous.

Anxiety syndromes, especially agoraphobia, are often manifestations of what we call LIAS (Lactate/Liver Induced Anxiety Syndrome). Anxiety is common in CFS patients simply because so many of the factors that cause or aggravate CFS also affect the liver. Increased lactate also causes muscular fatigue.

The aggravation of pre-existing pre-menstrual tension or the sudden onset of such problems is not uncommon or unexpected, especially if one considers the effect viruses can have on hormones and the endocrine glands. There are many types of pre-menstrual tension and alleviation of this condition depends on the characteristics of the syndrome.

GI symptoms
The GI symptoms, such as indigestion, abdominal bloating, constipation/diarrhoea, malabsorption, intestinal thrush and irritable bowel, are common symptoms of food allergies, or parasite or fungal infestations. The same symptoms can be caused by gastric viruses, abnormal gut flora (dysbiosis), candida overgrowth and inflammatory processes. Stool cultures, blood tests and a careful physical examination can often pinpoint the cause of these disturbances. Candida can be tested by measuring candida antibodies titres before and after antifungal medications.

Sensitivity to temperature changes
An abnormal sensitivity to temperature changes, especially cold extremities, may alert the diagnostician that the thyroid is malfunctioning and, after excluding APICHS, one must evaluate this possibility.

Lymph node swelling
Lymph node swelling (lymphadenopathy) is almost invariably associated with viral CFS as are sore throats and recurrent opportunistic infections such as *Candida albicans*.

Allergies and sensitivities
Inhalant allergies (dust mites, moulds/fungi, grasses, etc.), sensitivities to common chemicals (pesticides, pollution, car exhaust, etc.) and sinusitis, hay fever, asthma, post-nasal drip, excessive throat mucus, skin problems (eczema, dermatitis, etc.) are common. Testing for these presents a dilemma. First of all they may be temporary allergies which will improve or disappear once the underlying condition is taken care of. In such cases testing and treatment depends on the severity of the symptoms and whether or not the therapist thinks such allergies are hampering progress.

Even then, there is the additional dilemma of what test to do and how to interpret the results. In allergy tests, the immune system is asked to respond in a measurable way to a number of allergens (substances suspected of causing the allergy). It is simply impossible to test all the possible immune responses to one factor, even if we knew all the possible mechanisms, which we do not.

So tests are usually carried out for specific parts of our immune response. The most common ones are the IgE-mediated allergy responses. If the allergy is mediated via another factor (histamine, IgA, IgG, IgM, or whatever) then one will miss the allergy altogether. Measurements of oesinophils, IgA, IgG and IgM are therefore also carried out in many cases. They will indicate abnormalities but are not very useful for identifying the actual allergen.

As if this were not complex enough, there are many complications which can arise in the making, as well as the interpreting, of such measurements. For example, one may have a blood test called RAST (Radio Allergo Absorbent Test) for a great variety of foods, environmental factors, inhalants and toxic chemicals. These may prove negative.

It could be that a negative allergy test means that the patient has no allergy. On the other hand, it could be that the person is very allergic, so allergic in fact that immune responses are almost non-existent. Or it could be that the immune system is busy taking care of something else, perhaps a virus. Maybe an overload of chemicals has made a response impossible. There are tests to further elucidate these possibilities, such as the Cell Mediated Immunity Multitest.

These are just SOME of the interpretation problems we face every day.

The Candida antibodies test
For more on this test see Candida And CFS on p. 149.

Tiredness
There are many (all legitimate) causes of unusual and sometimes chronic tiredness. Any good therapist, however, will try to eliminate those before making a diagnosis of CFS.

A short list of these causes includes anaemia, liver disease, vitamin B12 deficiency, menopause, hypoglycaemia, diabetes, autoimmune disorder, kidney disease, hypothryoidism, multiple sclerosis, poor adrenal function, peripheral neuropathy, heart disease, cancer. As well, medically prescribed drugs, such as antihistamines, tranquillisers, analgesics, steroids, blood pressure medicines, diuretics, etc., can be the culprit.

In short, there are very few illnesses and medications that do not have at least the potential to make one feel unusually tired. Not to mention the myriad of emotional and lifestyle reasons.

And, of course, one can be tired because of poor nutrition or vitamin or mineral deficiencies.

VIRAL OR ENVIRONMENTAL?

There is little doubt that chemicals in our environment can affect our health in general and our resistance (immunity) in particular. So it is a bit like the chicken-or-the-egg question.

Nevertheless it is important to try to ascertain the cause or triggering factor in order to establish treatment priorities.

Environmental factors such as lifestyle, stress, poor nutrition, etc., are easily identifiable from questioning the patient and taking a careful history. The same applies to exposure to chemicals.

It is very important to understand that a SENSITIVITY to chemicals need not imply chemical overloading and, when such sensitivity occurs in the absence of high exposure, the possibility that a virus has caused this increased sensitivity must be thoroughly investigated.

Blood tests for levels of many chemicals are available and there are some tests that can show if some of these have affected the body. There are also urine analysis tests for several heavy metals as well as a number of 'allergy' tests which can show sensitivities to chemicals. These range from simple skin tests to intradermal end pointing, neutralisation, RAST and patch tests.

Apart from a thorough medical history and physical examination, which in itself may provide lots of clues, VIRAL factors are identifiable via blood tests which can screen patients for present as well as past viral infections. Usually this is the first step. In addition, sophisticated interpretation of these tests can tell the experienced diagnostician whether the original response to the virus was poor, if the attack is recurrent, if the virus is active or there is a chance of sporadic activity or reactivation and whether the virus may have caused a degree of immune suppression.

Immunological abnormalities are also recognisable, although there is considerable controversy over this. For example, some clinicians report that NK (natural killer cells) levels are low in patients with CFS, others find the number is usually higher than normal.

Viral CFS

The Viral Story

A great deal of human suffering can be traced to a humble life form that invades our cells, takes over and continues to thrive at our expense. This life form is the VIRUS.

It is clear by now that in some people CFS can be caused by a latent virus. In fact, the so-called 'Post Viral Syndrome' or Chronic Epstein Barr Virus Syndrome (CEBVS) is indistinguishable from CFS. It is also quite obvious that viruses will produce such effects only on susceptible individuals and history has shown that the number of such individuals is climbing steadily.

Viruses are no match for human cells. Physically they are many thousand times smaller. They are infinitely less complex and very much simpler. Yet their capacity for destruction once they enter a living body is nothing short of phenomenal. It's like a small child throwing a ball through the window of a skyscraper, and the whole building falling apart as a result.

But, in spite of many clues over the years, it was not until Professor Michael Oldstone, an immunologist and neuropharmacologist working at the Scripp Clinic and Research Foundation in La Jolla, California (USA), published a paper entitled 'Viral Alteration of Cell Functions' that many doctors started to suspect viruses as a factor in CFS.

Professor Oldstone clearly demonstrated how viruses can then act insidiously to alter cell function, neurotransmitter activity, hormone production and secretion, enzyme production, immune response and even myocardial contraction in such ways that they may be responsible for varied diseases such as growth retardation, diabetes, neurophsyiatric disorders, autoimmune diseases, blood sugar metabolism, aberrations and even heart disease. He discovered that persistent viral infection, even in the absence of symptoms, can alter the physiological functions of cells without destroying them because the cell's own life-sustaining functions are left alone so as to provide the virus with a comfortable home full of the sustenance it needs to survive and multiply.

Year after year we have seen influenza epidemics come and go. From Hong Kong to Europe, America, China and Australia — like pollution, the virus seems to know no boundaries. It is a safe bet that this year hundreds of thousands of individuals will suffer the flu, just as some did the year before and the year before that. Viral infections such as the flu are not only a matter of personal sufferings: they cost communities billions of dollars in lost production, accidents, health care, medications, etc.

In addition, viruses mutate. That is, they change constantly and each new variety can be more dangerous. At the beginning of this century an estimated 15 million people died as a result of a previously unknown type of flu virus.

In 1986, the Atlanta Center for Disease Control reported that viruses which are already present in normal, healthy organisms may become more virulent by repeated contact infections. Note that a contact infection can occur without anyone being aware of it — without the infection provoking any symptoms whatsoever (*Immunology Today,* Vol. 7, No. 1, 1986). One of the most difficult things for people to accept is that they may have a viral 'infection' without knowing it.

In 1986 Russian scientists confirmed the Atlanta studies by reporting that viral epidemics are more likely to occur when the young, with their immature immune systems and lowered immunocompetence, are infected by viral particles from their elders, incubate the virus, as it were, in their own bodies and then re-infect the elders.

There is considerable suspicion that the increasingly nefarious activity of viruses we are witnessing may be due not so much to the viruses themselves but to the increasing weakness of the organisms in which they take up residence. A healthy defence system is needed to keep viruses at bay.

There are countless types of viruses implicated in an enormous amount of human suffering. From viral hepatitis to viral arthritis and from the possibility of viral schizophrenia to cold sores, viruses of one kind or another have been implicated in all sorts of diseases. Recently we have seen the AIDS virus (HIV) raise its ugly head and there is every chance that more new viruses will strike in the future.

As you read these pages and become acquainted with recent scientific findings, you will understand that some types of CFS are in fact nothing more than a form of chronic viral illness, often caused by a specific virus known as the Epstein Barr virus, which is best known for causing glandular fever. Glandular fever is synonymous with infectious mononucleosis, or mono for short.

We have come to this conclusion after discovering the simple fact that viruses can affect almost any function of a living organism and often they can do that years, even decades, AFTER the original invasion has taken place. What is worse is that in many cases the affected individual is blissfully unaware that he/she has contacted the virus. The initial invasion often provokes no appreciable symptoms.

Viruses are incredibly small entities which lurk in a shadowy world poised somewhere between LIFE and NOT LIFE. They are a collection of genes (the basic information material which transmits personal characteristics from one generation to the next). They can pass back and forth from humans to animals, and vice versa.

When a virus invades a cell and takes over its running machinery, it does not take much to cause chaos. It is a little like tinkering with recording tape and splicing a bit from a Schubert sonata into a Beethoven symphony. The result would be a little like what happens when cancer strikes and is often similar to what goes on in the bodies of people affected by some viruses.

But a virus need not even go that far. It is quite capable of causing (the correct word is 'inciting') cancer on the spot, without any assistance. That is why people who harbour viruses, especially latent viruses, should do all they can to fight them off.

EPSTEIN BARR VIRUS

As we have seen, one of the most common viral offenders (although certainly not the only one) in CFS is the Epstein Barr virus (EBV). In underdeveloped countries, and perhaps in ancient times when hygiene was not a common virtue, EBV infected, and still infects, young people. When a child is infected by EBV, it rarely causes illness, but lies dormant, lurking in the vast majority of human beings. Like the infamous *Candida albicans* organism, EBV is opportunistic. And so many factors, including almost any other virus, can cause the dormant EBV to become active. Strangely enough, when we measure EBV and its effects it sometimes becomes clear that another virus was responsible for starting the illness — nevertheless, it is the EBV which eventually becomes reactivated and then causes the problem and, since the treatment for viral infections is similar irrespective of which virus started the problem, it makes sense to keep a close eye on the one that can be monitored closely.

Many viruses, such as the AIDS virus, are not smart at all in spite of their fearsome reputation. They kill the host. A little like someone invading your home, tying you up, then burning the house down while sitting in the armchair. Deadly yes — smart definitely not. It may, however, be a case of the virus being inexperienced, rather than stupid. After all, it is a relative newcomer on the scene and has a long way to go before it becomes street-wise like EBV, which EBV is — eminently so. EBV is a parasite and a clever one at that. It is as if it realises that its own survival depends on the survival of the host, so it does not kill you.

EBV commonly takes up permanent residence in a type of cell known as the B cell. It takes over and starts to act as if it owns the place. The viral population starts to proliferate. And it does this in the very cells that are responsible for making the antibodies that kill viruses.

Once installed, the virus may trigger off a full-blown attack of glandular fever or just a sore throat. (The throat soreness is caused by the fact that cells are torn open and leak viral particles. The nerves surrounding the throat's cells send alarm signals. PAIN!) Or it may make you feel unwell for a few days.

Irrespective of what it does cause, the virus remains in the cells forever. It 'hides' in the B cells and is capable of developing a special technique for shutting off its reproduction genes in order to make itself 'invisible' to the immune system. Very much like some modern airforce planes which have special anti-radar or radar-jamming equipment which renders them invisible to the enemy. In this way they are able to withstand even a perfectly normal immune system. That is one of the reasons why we always look for viruses in CFS patients and also one of the reasons why we are undeterred in our search for underlying 'causes' for

CFS in the absence of low immune capability. (Please remember: by the time the immune system has been measurably affected it may be too late.)

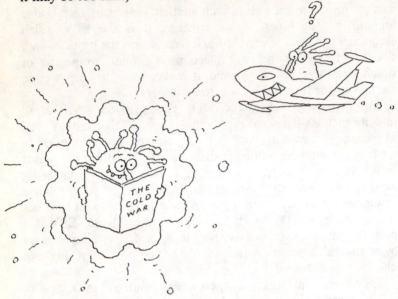

The virus-infected B cell doesn't stay in the dormant state forever. Perhaps it is switched on by triggering factors or perhaps it just likes to test the waters, as it were, to see how it would fare out in the wide open spaces of YOUR body.

Such 'megalomaniac' B cells turn into viral factories and start to spew thousands of viral particles (called capsids) into the blood. At this stage you start to make antibodies to these capsids (they are the ones we measure when we suspect an EBV-induced case of CFS).

Often the antibodies destroy the viral bits and that's that. You don't feel a thing. But sometimes the virus wins the battle against the antibodies. Perhaps you are run down, have a bacterial infection, candida or allergies. Perhaps you have unwittingly been exposed to a chemical.

From time to time one of the bits of the immune machinery that has the job of recognising viral particles, loses the battle and gives up. From that moment on the virus is immune to immunity.

I remember the story of a patient of mine who was quite happy and healthy. He took the family for a holiday in an expensive new hotel up north. They decided to go by car. Two twelve-hour days of driving in very hot weather. A few weeks after coming back, by car, the whole family started to feel unwell. They became so ill the mother hardly had the strength to get out of bed while her husband was fighting tooth and nail just to get to his job. Let alone do anything like hard work. The children just moaned, as children do, and looked sick. They even lost their appetites. A sure sign, as every parent knows, that something serious was afoot.

To make a long story short, the whole family had been exposed to the Epstein Barr virus some years before when one of the children had a touch of glandular fever. It provoked no symptoms in any of them. The hotel room they slept in up north had been heavily sprayed with chemicals to combat a plague of insects. The surrounding grass had been subjected to all sorts of insecticides to stop mosquitos and other bugs from annoying the guests. A blood test showed their blood had high levels of pesticides.

Perhaps their resistance was lowered by the stress of long car travel. Perhaps they had heated arguments on the road. Maybe they didn't get enough sleep. It is possible their car exhaust leaked a little. Who knows?

The result was that their defences were momentarily lowered and the Epstein Barr virus started to win the fight. The whole family got sick.

I got them well again, but it took some doing. Not the actual treatment; what took the doing was making them understand how a group of four, quite normal and reasonably healthy people could be struck by a devasting illness simply because of a holiday. Which they had taken to make them feel better in the first place.

But that's another story ...

From time to time one of the bits of the immune machinery that has the job of recognising viral particles, loses the battle and gives up. From that moment on the virus is immune to immunity.

No that's not a pun. It is a terrible fact with dire consequences for the host. YOU!

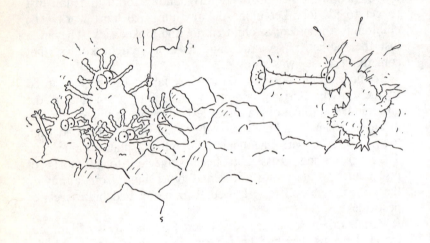

In the past few years, medical scientists have discovered several links between EBV and a variety of symptoms. In fact, these associations have often been noted in cases of chronic illness characterised by continuous relapses. (Sound familiar?) A list of eighteen symptoms attributed to EBV were outlined in the medical literature (*Annals of Internal Medicine,* January 1985) and guess what? They are almost the same as those that characterise CFS.

If you think AIDS is bad, please remember that numerically at least, chronic EBV is worse. I am not playing AIDS down. I just want to make a point. I know CFS is unlikely to kill you, or anyone. But many people struck by viral CFS live such miserable lives they often wish they were dead.

Be that as it may, people presenting with CFS were, until

recently, lumped together as sufferers of some sort of mystery illness, or they were told they were neurotics.

Those who were, unbeknown to them or their doctor, affected by EBV simply suffered the major symptom (chronic, inexplicable fatigue) along with any of the other symptoms. Some later developed cancers, or candida or severe neurological complications. Not realising these were only the FOOTPRINTS of EBV, each problem was attacked by a specialist in that area. Often with little success.

As I mentioned earlier, most people are exposed to EBV. Glandular fever, which is the full-blown illness sometimes caused by this virus, used to be known as the 'kissing disease'. There are other, perhaps less common routes of entry, such as skin cuts, sneezing, etc., but what you must keep in mind is that being in contact with and harbouring EBV does not necessarily mean anything.

It can spread to anyone near the infected individual. Then, even while dormant, it can reproduce. And then, when something causes the body's defences to weaken, it becomes active.

The available statistics show that the number of people afflicted with chronic EBV-type symptoms (remember these are practically indistinguishable from CFS) has been increasing steadily in the past fifteen years.

The chief of Internal Medicine at Peter Bent Brigham and Women's Hospital in Boston, Dr Anthony Kamaroff suggests that:

> Perhaps it is not the traditional EBV ... it could be a new mutant strain of EBV or it could be a whole new virus that somehow re-awakens old EBVs dormant in the patient's system. In fact, there is a suspect: human B-lymphotropic virus (HBLV), first identified in late 1986. Like EBV and chicken pox, it is in the herpes family of viruses, and it invades B cells, just as EBV does. HBLV could be making people sick all by itself and, in the process, re-awakening dormant EBV.

Dr Jesse A. Stoff is a physician with a great deal of experience in CFS in general and viral immunology in particular. He is also an expert on the EBV. This is how he explains it:

Once it is brought into contact with human B cells, EBV comes alive. The outer shell, or capsid, of the virus is shaped like a geodesic sphere and is composed of hollow, proteinaceous hexagons called capsomeres ... The Epstein Barr virus is unimaginably minute. Because the virus is actually smaller than a wavelength of light, it lives in a world without colour: everything is black and white. And yet, it displays extraordinary detail, geometrically complex and perfect, like a Herkimer diamond. That it is dangerous only adds spice to its beauty. Its capsomeres fit receptors on the membrane of the B cell, fusing with them as if the B cell were a loading dock built for its exclusive use. Once inside the host B cell, EBV sheds its capsomeres, and eventually grabs control of the cell's DNA, reprogramming it to make copies of the virus with a speed and sophistication even Xerox would envy. Alternatively the viral DNA can persist in a dormant state, awaiting the division and replication of the host cell, which will duplicate the EBV genes too, as hordes of new virus particles emerge from the cell nucleus ... The mere synthesis of such components as the viral capsid antigens kills the B cell ... The fatigue, fever and aches are not the result of a few infected cells dying. You feel awful because your body is mass producing antibodies and secreting mucus at an abnormally rapid pace. Persistent infections shift the body into maximum overdrive, triggering such complications as chronic inflammation. No, the virus does not always harm you directly, sometimes it is subtle and severe. Sometimes it deceives your own body into wearing itself down.

THE HISTORY OF EBV
The history of this virus has its origins in Uganda, Africa. It began when, in 1958, Dr Denis Burkitt discovered an unusual type of cancer of the immune system (lymphoma) that struck only the head and neck. The cancer was very fast, doubling in size every couple of days. It spread (metastasised) through the rest of the body quickly and was inevitably lethal. This condition was given the name of 'Burkitt's lymphoma'.

In 1964 a group of researchers at London's Middlesex Hospital (Anthony Epstein, B. G. Achong and Y. M. Barr) found some viral particles in the cells of Burkitt's lymphoma growths. That is how this virus got its name.

Later, it was shown that EBV antibodies are present in all children with this type of cancer. But then the same antibodies were also found in the blood of ALL HEALTHY children aged four or less. The only difference was that those afflicted with the cancer had much higher titre counts than the healthy ones.

No one is absolutely sure what this association means except for the fact that some people are obviously responding to EBV in special ways. The strong suspicion exists that the bodies of certain individuals become a sort of viral factory and that there is some sort of two-way traffic in the effects of some illnesses and the EBV. Reported cases of ankolysing spondilitis have been found to be triggered by this virus, the disease then weakening the body further while the virus sends the whole immune system into a state of confusion.

Then it was discovered that EBV is part of a wider group of viruses, the so-called herpes family. Other members of the herpes virus family include genital herpes, chicken pox and the cytomegalovirus (CMV). Recently another herpes virus, human herpes virus 6 (HHV-6) has been implicated in CFS.

It is known that EBV can be oncogenic, meaning it can cause different kinds of cancers. It is also known that EBV weakens the mechanisms by which the body keeps tabs on wayward cells that may become cancer cells. One such cancer, known as nasopharyngeal carcinoma, because it occurs in the pharynx and the back of the nose, is prevalent in some parts of China. The children in those regions invariably contract EBV early in life, without showing any signs or symptoms of infection. In some of these children, the virus, after waiting for years, even decades, for some reason wakes up and leads to the development of cancer. Yet after trying as hard as they could, researchers failed to provoke the growth of cancer cells after exposing them to EBV in their labs. Something was missing. Something that interacted with EBV and turned it on, as it were. In 1987 the puzzle was solved. The Chinese living in the areas with a high incidence of both EBV and nasopharyngeal carcinoma used a common Chinese herbal folk remedy containing compounds known as phorbolesters. (Phorbolesters are widely used in some wood paints and other commercial applications in many countries.)

When the EBV-laden cells were exposed to phorbolesters, the virus incited the growth of cancer cells! It was discovered that EBV sometimes needed a 'promoter' to turn on its fully blown nastiness. Therefore we now understand that while EBV itself may or may not directly cause anything at all, its very presence in the body makes it a recipe for disaster should one be exposed to promoting or triggering factors.

Now you should clearly understand that 'official' pronouncements which claim that such-and-such a chemical is 'safe' because it took kilograms of it before it killed a laboratory rat, and therefore 'normal' exposure can't possibly harm you or your family, are nonsense when one considers the many and very subtle ways in which chemicals can act as promoters or triggers. Sophisticated tests, or rather the interpretation of some tests, can make us suspicious. When we do have suspicions, we can change the course of our therapy and make further investigations to confirm or disprove our feelings.

As you will learn in the section on What You Can Do to Help Yourself (see p. 132), we are poised on the threshold of being able to determine if your home or personal environment is a source of potentially dangerous chemicals. We will be able to identify and measure the chemicals and, if necessary, check whether there are any of those chemicals in your body.

We know that stress, chemicals of all kinds, other infections such as candida, and a host of other factors may directly or indirectly cause reactivation of the Epstein Barr virus. That is one of the reasons why testing for Epstein Barr virus (EBV) in cases of Chronic Fatigue Syndrome is so important, even if the problem is caused by another factor, or even another virus such as HLBV (Human B lymphotropic virus) or HHV-6 (Human herpes 6 virus).

Please do not misunderstand what I have just told you. Do not assume that if you have EBV in your body you are automatically going to get CFS or cancer or even anything at all. On the other hand, do not assume that if you have had a viral infection sometime in the past and are now a CFS sufferer, that this means that Chronic EBV infection is *the* cause of your Chronic Fatigue Syndrome. It may not be. It is not in many, many cases of CFS.

Diagnosis

The diagnosis of virally induced CFS is either difficult or comparatively easy, depending on circumstances. Unlike the diagnosis of chemical CFS, which relies heavily on exclusion of other causes and a comprehensive history of the circumstances involved in the onset of the problems, viral CFS can be diagnosed mostly by blood tests.

There are certain problems with the interpretation of lab results and unfortunately there are still some doctors out there that are not familiar with them.

THE TITRES — 'VIRAL FOOTPRINTS'

The reason we always measure EBV parameters, and spend a lot of time interpreting the results of each case, is that any form of EBV activity can be a sign of something acting as a trigger or promoter, which we then painstakingly look for. The tests measure the 'footprints' left by the virus. There are only a few pathologists in Australia who are able to provide your doctor with a full Epstein Barr viral screening.

When your doctor sends your blood to a pathologist for an EBV screening, one of the most important diagnostic factors will be the 'titres' against viral capsids particles called 'viral capsid antibodies' (VCA) (see p. 245).

When antibodies to a specific virus or other 'enemies' are measured, their presence tells your doctor that you have been in contact with the EBV. Even if you have been exposed five, ten or twenty years ago, the test will find out. This in itself is not necessarily a problem. As we've seen, most people have been exposed to the virus during their lifetime and most, if not all, people would show some such sign of earlier contact — just like most people have SOME *Candida albicans* organisms in the body, yet not everybody suffers the consequences.

We can also find out just how much you may have been, or are, affected by EBV by diluting your blood serum in a watery solution, called saline, and repeating the dilution at the rates of 1 part serum to 10 parts saline, then 1 to 20, 1 to 40, 80, 160, 320, etc. The presence of viral antibodies when the solution is greatly diluted means that a strong infection has occurred and this information is then related to other findings to make a diagnosis.

In general, the titres of viral antibodies give us a measurement of the way the body is fighting the battle. We may consider there is a problem when the VCA count is 160 or above (other specialists suggest a problem only if 640 or over) but of course each lab will have its own parameters. That is one reason why it is important always to use the same lab when investigating such matters.

Then there is the usual controversy over the interpretation of levels and their meaning.

As always, lab test results must be measured against the doctor's personal knowledge of the patient and his/her clinical judgement and assessment of priorities.

Variations

The actual values of viral titres (IgG, VCA, etc.) can, and do, vary considerably during the course of the illness, and even between individuals. When taken at any particular point, they are nothing more than a snapshot of the virus's footprints at any one time, and this alone cannot be used for an accurate diagnosis.

In his book *Chronic Fatigue Syndrome,* which deals thoroughly and almost exclusively with Epstein Barr-induced CFS, Dr Jesse A. Stoff put it this way:

> The antibodies to EBV which play a key role in putting the virus into remission and keeping it there, can be almost undetectable, initially, in those who have been chronically ill for a long time. As the immune system recovers, these antibodies will appear and remain for several months, or even years, after the virus has been beaten.

SYMPTOMS

During the acute stage the symptoms will be more characteristically those of a severe flu: fatigue, sore throat, fever, aches and pains, headaches, perhaps sweating, with some swollen glands and tenderness or even swelling of liver and spleen. Sometimes a liver function test will show some abnormalities.

When there is viral re-activation, and during the acute stages of such re-activation, most of these signs and symptoms will recur.

Even after the acute stage has passed, most, if not all of the above tend to persist but other complications may set in: blood sugar disturbances (hypoglycaemia), allergies and opportunistic infections such as candida, etc.

If this state of affairs is allowed to continue, people begin to suffer more and more mental, mood or neurological problems, especially with memory and concentration problems, depression and anxiety. At this stage, allergy tests, such as RAST, may become positive.

Unfortunately, sometimes things get even worse. At that point, almost anything can happen. According to medical experts such diverse organs as the ovaries, the thyroid, the pancreas, the brain and, of course, the immune system may be severely affected. Autoimmune diseases can also occur.

Clues may be: abnormal thyroid function tests (low T4s, high TSH); allergy tests are negative, in spite of full-blown allergic symptoms; various immunoglobulins may be affected (low or elevated IgGs and low IgAs); the T helpers:T suppressors (T4:T8) ratio may fall; natural killer cells may suddenly increase or decrease; and the adrenals (the glands responsible for our stress response) may become less efficient (serum cortisol levels may show a flattening of the daily time curve).

DON'T RELY ON THE TEST RESULTS

Because viruses can affect just about any organ and system in the body, one must consider all the clinical aspects of the patient's health. One problem is worth further consideration.

If one only counts the titres, one may be misled. Titres can climb dramatically during treatment, and may signal an abatement of the disease progress. In such cases the titres will increase as the patient improves. This state of affairs will be followed by a steady decline in titres, as the patient improves further following the immune system's successful attack.

The Liver

One of the primary targets of EBV and other viruses (as well as some non-viral organisms such as the toxoplasmosis organism), the liver's role in metabolism and immunity is often the first to suffer. Many EBV patients develop sub-acute hepatitis, CFS and depression.

One of the most important first-line defences is provided by a group of cells called *macrophages* (from the Greek for 'large-eaters'). They originate in the bone marrow and are then in the form of *monocytes*. They become macrophages once they enter the bloodstream and take up residence in various tissues. They are large scavengers which attack enemies much like the blobs in some arcade and home television games such as Pac Man, Space Invaders, etc.

There are many 'colonies' of these 'big eaters' in various parts of the body and they are collectively known as the 'reticuloendothelial system' (RES). Just like the transport department has buses, taxis, trams and private as well as commercial vehicles dispersed all over a State or country but is still regarded as a 'system'.

Interestingly, macrophages, or the RES if you prefer, are particularly abundant in the digestive tract, the spleen, the lungs, connective tissues and the nervous system. But by far the greatest concentration of this formidable army of big eaters is in the liver. Here they are referred to as 'Kupffer cells' in honour of their discoverer. They make up some 10 per cent of the entire liver's mass and their main job is to keep the liver clear of viruses.

A little dumb, macrophages are unable to recognise individual viruses; they gobble up only clumps of such enemies after they have been identified and 'tied up' by antibodies. They then send signals to antibodies about the presence of foreigners so more antibodies can tie up more viruses. Viruses thus bound to antigen-antibody complexes are immediately dispatched to the liver where they have to filter through the RES network of macrophages, which then eats up the lot: viruses, antibodies, the whole clump!

That sounds like a good job; and indeed it is. But there are drawbacks. The average human body creates several million new immune cells and antibodies each day. Even if one is blessed with perfect health, chances are his/her body harbours millions of viruses. And there are thousands of different kinds of viruses. At best, scientists have identified some 10 per cent of them. So, as you can well imagine, portions of the immune system continue to gather up antigen-antibodies and form more and more of these 'lumps'. And they will grow in size. They will double up. Then double up again unless the macrophages in the liver (the Kupffer cells of the RES system) can maintain a frantic gobbling-up pace. If the liver defences are short-handed, or a little slower than they should be, two things can happen. First of all more and more antibodies form complexes and are thus removed from circulation where they are desperately needed to catch more roaming viruses. Secondly, the lumps can grow so big that they actually block the kidneys on their way out via the urine.

Now that you know all this, you will begin to appreciate that the liver of CFS sufferers must be thoroughly investigated. Iris diagnosis, Chinese pulse diagnosis, blood tests, physical examination, lifestyle and eating habits questionnaires, medical history, a full knowledge of all drugs taken for whatever reason in the past — anything at all that will give information about the patient's liver functions is very important.

How really important it is to look after your liver will become even clearer when I tell you a few more facts which also point to the intertwining of viral and chemical CFS.

In addition to trying to keep you clear of viral dangers, the liver also plays a similar role with bacteria and pathogenic fungi such as *Candida albicans*. That is one of the reasons we always treat any existing candida infection vigorously, irrespective of its apparent severity, or lack of it.

Then consider the fact that your liver has to detoxify, break down and dispose of most drugs. Many, if not the majority of pharmaceutical drugs prescribed for serious ailments, tend to damage the liver somewhat (hepatotoxicity) — this is the reason why CFS sufferers should avoid drugs as far as possible.

Then the liver also has the job of taking care of any alcohol you may drink. Apart from the fact that alcohol itself can compromise the functions of a liver, this organ has to do an additional job if you have a viral problem AND drink at the same time. So alcohol is a big no-no for CFS sufferers.

Finally, please note that the liver also takes care of the majority of xenobiotics and other chemicals that enter your body through the skin, inhalation or ingestion. If you hang freshly dry-cleaned clothes in your wardrobe overnight, if you use a self-service petrol station, if you work near a photocopier, if you use paint solvents, indeed, if you sleep in a house that has been freshly painted, recently carpeted or has had pest fumigation, chances are SOME

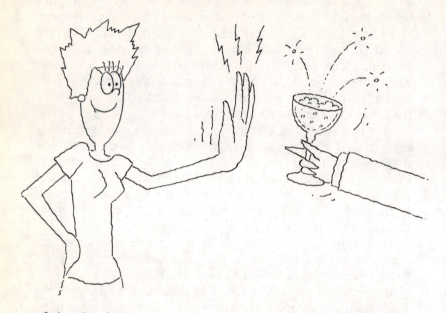

of the chemicals are in your blood. And the liver may already have a full-time job coping with that. Then you add alcohol and are unfortunate enough to have your EBVs re-activated!

'How much can a koala bear?' is one of the funniest inscriptions I have seen on a T-shirt. 'How much can a liver bear?' should be written on a 5 x 2 metres banner in every CFS sufferer's home.

Chemical CFS

Your Environment

During the last half of this century our influence on the environment has gone from bad to worse. In addition, some things have changed. While the deterioration of our environment continues, humans 'tighten up' their homes and workplaces more and more. Air-conditioning, gas heaters, insulation, tightly shut doors, windows and buildings are now commonplace. They do keep us cool in the summer and warm in the winter and they do shut out much noise and save on electricity, thus helping the conservation of our natural resources. But too many individuals have paid and are paying a high price for this state of affairs.

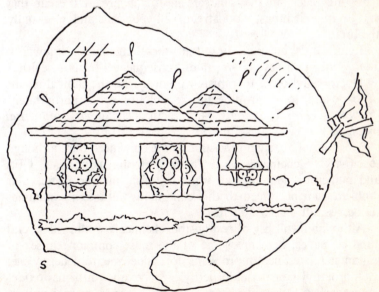

A quick glimpse at the common sources of chemicals will show you that these abound in all types of inhabited buildings. They allow chemicals to leak into the air and we breathe them. This leaking process is sometimes called 'outgassing'. This is not as strange as you may think. If you have a bunch of flowers on the table, the chances are that some molecules from the flowers are *in* you. All things continuously age, rust, break down, deteriorate and undergo oxidation. During this process molecules of the breakdown float away from the source and into the air you breathe. That's why you can smell the flowers. On the other hand, some chemicals cannot be smelled. Yet they can kill you. That is how people die from carbon monoxide poisoning. They can't smell it! Chemicals can enter your lungs, from where they inevitably enter the bloodstream.

Chances are your car interior has lots of plastic components, such as a urethane steering wheel. Leave the car in the hot sun and this will cause extra outgassing as the plastic surfaces become hot and begin to disintegrate, ever so slightly. Drive by an outdoor showroom for new cars on a hot day. You may notice a slight film on the inside of the windscreens. That film is composed of chemical particles which outgass from the plastics and find a resting place on the windscreen. If you are in the car they end up in your lungs, bloodstream, all your cells and, eventually, the brain.

Evidence is accumulating that these chemicals, known as *xenobiotics,* can have far-reaching consequences for our health.

Doctors and other therapists who deal with the clinical results of exposure to environmental xenobiotics are, appropriately, known as *clinical ecologists* or practitioners of *environmental medicine.*

Most, if not all, such practitioners are convinced that, although sensitivity to chemicals varies greatly among individuals, CFS and numerous neurological, immunological and neuromuscular problems can be traced to this continuous, although sometimes subtle, assault on our system.

Although a full list of responsible chemicals would fill several hundred pages, here are some of the most common causes of buildings-related health problems: formaldehyde; toluene; xylene; trichloroethylene; perichloroethylene; hexane; nitrous oxide; ozone; carbon monoxide; carbon dioxide; alkanes; petrochemicals and other hydrocarbons.

One of the problems with chemical sensitivity is that one never knows, at least at the onset, whether the sensitivity is caused by unsuspected exposure to a large amount, a long term exposure to a small amount or a sudden hypersensitivity brought on by something else which has depleted our resistance. And then it could be a virus, or stress, or something else.

Yet so many people ask: 'Why me?' And: 'Why all of a sudden when I have touched, eaten, drunk or breathed the same things all my life without problems?' The answer is, of course, that when your resistance is lowered you may become allergic (intolerant) to some food that never gave you any problems or you may become ill when exposed to a common chemical your body tolerated reasonably well until then.

It is a very simple, yet much misunderstood problem. Try to think of it in this way. You have a circle of friends and acquaintances among which are individuals whom you do not particularly like but can put up with easily. Then you have a bad day. And on that day, of all days, you get a cold, have urgent problems at work — and your car won't start. Outside it is pouring with rain.

The chances are that your social resistance will be somewhat lowered. Perhaps to the point where you can't stand the chattering of an acquaintance you never worried much about. Perhaps someone's music will seem too loud, even irritating to you. Under such circumstances you may well behave rather anti-socially and turn someone from a neutral acquaintance into an enemy.

All of a sudden you are hypersensitive to previously tolerated people or events! In exactly the same way, if your resistance is lowered, you may become allergic to some food that never gave you any problems and you may become ill when exposed to a common chemical your body tolerated until then.

Or you may become intolerant to substances in your environment that sometimes you can't even smell, let alone see or taste! For example, if you work in an office, chances are there is a photocopier somewhere. One of the many chemicals that can outgas from photocopiers is trichloroethylene (TCE). TCE is used in dry cleaning fluids, carpet shampoos, some floor polishes and some furniture polishes. You breathe some. It enters the blood. TCE can cause mental confusion, fatigue, numbness and tingling sensations, headaches, dizziness, muscle cramps and other symptoms.

Your home may not be as safe as you think, either! Chemicals are present to some degree in the vast majority of offices and very many homes. Many chemicals are lipid-soluble, which means they can get into cell membranes and the brain (the brain is one of the most lipid organs), causing all sorts of symptoms, including depression, anxiety and exhaustion.

General practitioners tend to classify patients as having emotional problems or psychiatric problems when they can't find a physical cause for the presenting physical symptoms. Or they say that it is psychosomatic or 'all in the mind'. Some of these people come to us because they know, or feel, that there is nothing wrong with their mind and would like to continue searching for physical reasons for their problems. However, although not in the *mind,* a lot of their problems can be in the *brain.*

The facts are that human brains are susceptible to an incredible array of factors which can alter their biochemistry in ways capable of reducing even the sanest person to a sociopathic moron. Just spend some time in a pub around closing time in most cities and you will see how the introduction of a relatively simple, natural chemical (alcohol) into the brain can dramatically alter human behaviour.

Stop and think about it for a minute or two and you will realise that if a normal, intelligent human being can be made to alter his or her behaviour so profoundly as to 'be' another person just by adding a few drops of alcohol to the brain, then adding other, often toxic and very unnatural, chemicals to the brain, or altering the balance between the various chemicals which control brain functions in general and the brain cells' communication in particular, may produce similar alterations in behaviour.

As a case in point, consider the experience of Dr Sherry Rogers, a Fellow of the American College of Allergy and Immunology, a Fellow of the American Board of Family Practice, a Fellow of the American Academy of Environmental Medicine and a member of the American College of Occupational Medicine, who practises in New York and works at the Community General Hospital there — hardly a person to dismiss lightly. Dr Rogers is normally a healthy, happy person with a good sense of humour who enjoys her work, her husband and her travels. She has this to say:

I was lecturing in China and we registered in a recently refurbished hotel. Within minutes (of entering the hotel room) I was nasty, negative, sarcastic and crying over nothing. My husband immediately recognised what was happening, took me outside and, after twenty minutes outdoors, I was happy and laughing again.

And no, Dr Rogers was not drunk. Dr Rogers was not mad. Dr Rogers had not just fallen victim of some mysterious disease. She did not need tranquillisers, either. What she needed was fresh, clean air — unpolluted by paint fumes, cleansing solvents, plastic outgassings and aerosol sprays which permeated the rooms.

Poor Dr Rogers suffers from a condition she treats very often in her patients. We call it TBS for the Toxic Brain Syndrome. In the last twenty years I have seen and treated thousands of patients from all over Australia who suffered profound changes in their physical and mental health as a consequence of their hypersensitivities, intolerance or, if you prefer, allergies to commonly used chemicals and environmental pollutants or airborne moulds and dust particles. In some cases these unfortunate people find themselves on the edge of insanity and, aided and abetted by inexperienced medical practitioners, begin to question their own lucidity and capacity for rational thinking after they are repeatedly told that 'it's all in your mind'.

Fortunately there are ways to diagnose both chemical overloading (chemical CFS) and chemical hypersensitivity. The first is done with blood tests, the second with a variety of techniques. Probably the most successful, if controversial, is the one used by Dr Rogers herself, now finding its way to Australia. Called 'provocation-neutralisation', the technique not only ferrets out the responsible chemicals, but often can be used successfully to 'neutralise' the sensitivity with a series of injections.

To the claims that the effects may be 'all in the mind' Dr Rogers answers by describing how she has successfully treated horses, and asthmatic horses at that, with this technique. She filmed the procedure and published the report *(Clinical Ecology,* Vol. 5, No. 4, 1988).

There are five basic principles in environmental medicine, according to Dr Mark Donohoe:

1. *Total body load* explains why reactions vary from day to day, are never the same, and can vary from person to person.
2. *Adaptation* or *masking* can occur whereby the body gets 'used to' a toxin and adjusts itself for the time being. Meanwhile, accumulation proceeds, the body is stressed and somewhere along the line an apparent sudden deterioration occurs.
3. *Biochemical individuality* and *individual susceptibility* mean that no two people will get exactly the same symptoms from the same exposure. Likewise, people with similar symptoms can have different causes.
4. *Bipolarity:* a stimulation phase followed by a down. The stimulation can be misinterpreted as good and the individual may become addicted to the stimuli. He/she learns to repeat exposure or ingestion in order to avoid the 'down' phase. Very much like an alcoholic.
5. The *spreading phenomenon,* which occurs when the pathways used to dispose of a toxin become more overloaded, damaged or depleted so that one becomes more and more sensitive to new factors and to lower doses of the same toxins. The ability to tolerate toxins decreases.

ENVIRONMENTAL MEDICINE

These conclusions underline the fact that there is probably no branch of medical science that is more pivotal to the maintenance of good health than environmental medicine. Environmental medicine (also known as clinical ecology) deals with the increasing number of people affected by the continuing deterioration of our environment so that they tend to become poisoned by, or sensitive/allergic to, more and more substances, be they common foods or chemicals.

There is little doubt in my mind that the problem is getting worse and that we will see more and more people becoming ill because of environmental pollution. And because some of the most profound effects of xenobiotics (foreign chemicals) may take many years to cause symptoms and because they generally weaken the organism's resistance and pave the way for degenerative diseases, environmental medicine deals today with problems that will confront most health workers tomorrow. For this reason it is sometimes called 'tomorrow's medicine today'.

We have recently witnessed the public outcry caused by the pollution of city beaches. It was only after several well-known people revealed how they suffered recurring infections and bouts of ill health after swimming and after scientists described the toxicity and carcinogenicity (potential to cause cancer) of many chemicals found in our water, and the fishes that live there, that something started to be done about it. That is, after people have become well informed. Alas! The same is not yet happening in regard to the thousands of toxic chemicals we breathe, drink, eat and touch in the course of our daily lives.

Natural/holistic forms of medicine in general, and naturopathy in particular, have always maintained that orthodox medicine fails to look at the real causes of illness because it is too preoccupied with alleviating symptoms. It is time that we realised that toxic chemical overloads are probably one of the most basic 'causes' of human disease in the latter part of the twentieth century and that doing something about our environment represents the ultimate form of prevention.

Disease in general can be considered an individual's reaction to assaults on his/her external or internal environment (by bacteria, viruses, stresses, pollution, chemicals or whatever), modified by that individual's susceptibility. It is obvious that, unlike our ability to choose who we marry or what we wear, we are all forced to breathe the same air, drink the same water pollutants and be exposed to the same chemicals — whether we like it or not.

When the accumulation of these chemicals exceeds our individual capacity to detoxify ourselves (via liver detoxification and antioxidant activity) or when one is particularly susceptible to the effects of these chemicals, then our general capacity to deal with the myriad of bacteria, viruses, illnesses and stresses which confront us daily can diminish alarmingly. Only at that point do we become ill.

Any disease, however, is only able to take hold because our natural resistance, our defence mechanisms, have become inadequate. While diagnosing and treating the illness is of paramount importance, it must be obvious that finding, correcting or treating the underlying cause is the only way in which we can assure ourselves of an effective cure. I have lost count by now of the patients I have seen who have great difficulties in losing their allergies, candida and other opportunistic infections or ridding themselves of persistent viral diseases, such as glandular fever or chronic fatigue, simply because they are chemically overloaded.

Clear evidence of the increasing 'weakness' and lowered resistance to disease can be seen in every doctor's surgery, every allergist's office and every nutritionist's rooms. Indeed, the number of people suffering the consequences of such impaired resistance (allergies, candida, malnutrition, obesity, cancers, CFS, psychiatric problems, alcoholism, recurrent viral and bacterial illnesses) has increased alarmingly in the past decade. What is even more terrifying is that where once we used to see mostly older patients affected by these ills, nowadays the proportion of young people presenting themselves is mounting steadily.

It is not always easy to avoid toxic chemicals. Hexachlorobenzene (HCB), which is alleged to be carcinogenic and known to reduce immunocompetence, is banned in Australia. However, blood levels of Australians show them to be still heavily contaminated. Some of us believe that HCB is still being used to spray grains in this country. The existence of huge stockpiles may cause this practice to continue for another decade. Yet more and more people are urged to eat complex carbohydrates (grains) every day: 'Good for constipation!', 'It will lower cholesterol!', 'The only way to prevent heart disease!' urge the daily headlines. What about the possibility that it may increase the chemical load and contribute to cancer? What about the thousands that become allergic to these grains?

Eating more meat is even worse, considering the chemicals found in our animal foods. The problems created by all this are staggering but at least we can warn people as to where the invisible, subtle pollution occurs. We can explain to them that carpets, glues, particleboard, plywood, perfumes, dishwashing detergents, copying paper and tobacco, just to name a few, are often impregnated with formaldehyde and that this chemical is suspected of causing havoc with our immune systems. Or that having long, hot showers, especially after swimming for hours in a chlorinated pool, will increase your chlorine load perhaps beyond tolerable levels. Swimming in the sea can also be quite hazardous these days, so what is one to do? We tell our patients to use saltwater pools or swim in unpolluted areas. Then have only short showers with lukewarm water or else find a showerhead filter that will remove chlorine.

We also advise that styrene plastic cups filled with hot tea and lemon may poison them and wrapping food in plastic will contaminate it. We urge them not to use deodorants with aluminium or use bleached nappies for their babies. Phthalic acid esters (phthalates) are commonly used to make plastic softer, so that it can be wrapped around foods and they can make up as much as 50 per cent of the mass of a PVC container. Phthalates can leach from containers, are fat soluble and can be absorbed through the skin. They damage the liver, are classed as teratogenic (can harm a foetus) and mutagenic (can cause mutations). In mammals, they may induce liver or testicular cancer. They 'use up' a considerable amount of antioxidants.

We warn our patients that water must be filtered, and not just with a carbon filter. Reverse osmosis AND a filter must be used, or else water should be distilled.

The world we live in is full of chemicals — so what is one to do? The scientists who deal with the problems these chemicals cause are called *clinical ecologists*. They diagnose and treat the medical (clinical) or psychiatric effects of environmental allergic-chemical overloads in human beings.

ENVIRONMENTAL ILLNESS

Chemical overloading, chemical hypersensitivity, heavy metal toxicity, mould/mycotoxin poisoning, severe allergic illness ... whatever one chooses to call these problems, they all add up to the same thing: environmental illness.

The environment, meaning what you breathe, eat, drink, touch, feel, relate to, etc., is unfriendly, stressful and perhaps toxic to you. It may be that you are different from other people and are affected by factors which others can shrug off. It may be that a long-forgotten viral attack has left you weaker and more easily affected. It could be that your emotional state or personal life is so stressful that your resistance has been lowered to the point where all sorts of normally encountered substances make you ill, but leave others around you unscathed. It could be one, or a combination of very many factors. There are many reasons why one person will become ill as a result of exposure to chemicals while someone else may retain good health.

The most common points to remember are:

- Chemical sensitivity or overloading can happen to anyone, any time and, when it occurs, any organ, any body system can be affected, directly or indirectly.
- The onset of symptoms may be gradual, insidious, or may develop suddenly. Many factors influence an individual's susceptibility to chemical exposure. Among them are:
    genetic-hereditary factors
    nutritional status
    total body load
    biochemical individuality
    immunological individuality
    the degree of adaptation, or masking
    the biological activity of the chemical
    the length and degree of exposure
    general and emotional health at the time of exposure
    previous exposure events
    viral, bacterial or fungal infections
    emotional or physical trauma, that is, surgery, accident, etc.

Are You Tired, or Toxic?

That is the question put by one of the world's leading authorities on environmental illness, the diagnosis and treatment of chemically related problems, and the body's detoxification (detox) pathways.

Dr Sherry Rogers came to Australia in 1989 to deliver a series of lectures, which I attended, teaching Australian environmental doctors all she could about the subject. In addition, I have attended several international conferences on CFS and related subjects in Europe and America in the past few years, and I spent some time at Dr William Rea's Environmental Center in Dallas (Texas, USA) learning about his diagnostic and treatment procedures. That trip included a visit to ACCU—CHEM, the United States' leading laboratory for chemical analysis. From all these symposia, conferences, meetings and Dr Sherry Rogers' many lectures, scientific papers, books and other publications, I have compiled the following report.

THE BODY DETOXIFICATION SYSTEM
The body possesses a unique system that, until recently, medical science has neglected to acknowledge. In fact, most medical textbooks of the 1970s and 1980s do not even mention it in terms of environmental illness. This detox system exists in every cell of the body.

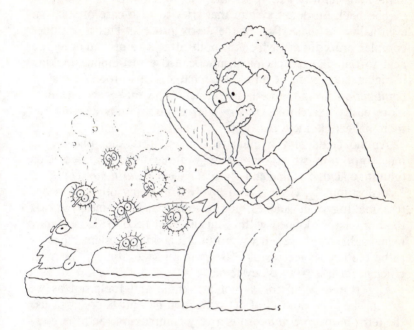

Research into the subject received a great impetus when space medicine found it had to resolve problems arising from chemical contamination from outgassing materials in space capsules. Other scientists studied how the body protects itself against the onslaught of an ever-increasing number of chemicals (xenobiotics) which permeate our environment.

The body has to process, metabolise or change practically everything that enters it. Most xenobiotics are changed into safer, or less toxic, substances so they can be excreted without poisoning the body further. Like any system however, the detox system can be inefficient, overloaded, damaged and, on occasions, swamped, so that it almost comes to a standstill.

There are two phases of the detox process. Phase One occurs inside cells and involves reactions like oxidation, reduction, hydrolysis, etc. These terms simply refer to the process by which the composition of chemicals is changed in specific ways (removing or adding electrons or hydrogen atoms, etc.). However, once the poison starts to exit from your body, it may do some damage on its way out. To the kidneys, for example.

The back-up detox system that tries to take care of such an eventuality is Phase Two of the detox process. This is a rather complex procedure by which the body attaches a protein or amino acid to the changed chemical, now called a metabolite, making it bigger and giving it an electric charge. This process is called *conjugation,* from the Latin for 'attach'. This makes the chemical more easily excretable via the bile or stools, thus keeping the more delicate kidneys out of it.

Amino acids play a major role in all this, and one of the most important is one combination of three different amino acids (glutamic acid, cysteine and glycine) called *glutathione (GSH).*

Unfortunately, GSH is also involved in many other processes (the making of hormones, genetic materials, enzymes, etc.). If the body is overloaded with chemicals that need GSH, less may be available for those other important functions. Cysteine appears to be the key to successful GSH synthesis and ability. The most efficient form is N-acetyl-cysteine.

Unfortunately all this is not as simple and foolproof as we would like. The process of detoxification (scientists prefer to use the term *biotransformation*) is a very complex one and the body has to choose between many possible metabolites in which to change the chemical. Sometimes it chooses the wrong one and the body ends up with a metabolite that is more toxic than the chemical we started with.

Then there is another problem. The body has to choose, from so many available pathways, the most suitable at the time. Because detox involves enzymes and because there are innumerable enzymes, each highly specific for one reaction only, when the body is overloaded with one particular chemical, it may not have enough reserves of one of the special enzymes needed at the time. Because no other enzyme will do, the xenobiotic continues its path of destruction. Many, if not all, the enzymes involved in detox need a particular vitamin or

CHEMICAL CFS

mineral in order to work. They are practically paralysed if there is a deficiency.

It is quite possible to be affected by xenobiotics simply because you are, unknowingly, deficient in a key mineral or because your body has unusual requirements for that one nutrient. In that case it is called a 'dependency' as against a deficiency. Remember, each person is biochemically unique.

When, for whatever reason, there are more chemicals in the body than the detox system can handle, damage can occur. Often to the mitochondria — the so-called powerhouse of the cells. By the time the detox system catches up with any backlog, some damage may have already occurred. Now you know why sometimes you do not feel better as soon as you take all the supplements prescribed. They may just stop FURTHER damage from occurring.

A blockage, or slow down, of detox activity can cause other problems. The chemical that can't get through may damage you, but so will all the chemicals that follow — those that you are exposed to all the time without knowing. These, in turn, may cause further damage to the detox system, starting a chain reaction that can lead to all sorts of health problems — including cancer. CFS patients at this stage feel like they have fallen apart.

The pathway your body chooses to get rid of a chemical depends on what enzymes are available, the level of nutrients (vitamins, minerals, amino acids, etc.) on hand, the total load at the time, the degree of damage to the detox pathways that may have been caused by other chemicals before you even became aware that there is such a thing as CFS.

DETOX PATHWAY BOTTLENECKS

In Phase One many xenobiotics are first changed into alcohols, which then must be metabolised to aldehydes. Only from the aldehyde stage can the chemical be then safely excreted as an acid via the urine. Alcohol dehydrogenase is the enzyme involved in converting the alcohol to its aldehyde.

Please understand two important things:

1. The fact that women CFS sufferers seem to outnumber males and the fact that their symptom clusters appear to include more 'nervous' symptoms is not necessarily a figment of

chauvinistic physicians; it may simply be due to the fact, discovered only late in 1989, that females tend to have LESS alcohol dehydrogenase enzymes than males.
2   Australian and other Anglo-Saxon populations seem to have a disproportionately high occurrence of CFS. They also tend to drink more alcohol, particularly without eating at the same time. This appears to be an important factor. When there is alcohol in the system, the body uses its supplies of alcohol dehydrogenase to break the alcohol down rather than toxic chemicals. It is, therefore, imperative that CFS sufferers learn to avoid alcohol at all cost. And that is not the only reason (see The Liver pp. 87). It is a similar story for chronic candida victims too (see Candida and CFS pp. 149).

Phase Two bottlenecks also occur whenever there are not enough antioxidants.

HERE TODAY, GONE TOMORROW
One of the most frustrating experiences for an environmental doctor is to be faced by a patient who is clearly bombed out by chemicals but tells you something along these lines:

'Impossible! If chemical X was a problem, how come nothing happened when I was exposed to it on some days, while at other times I felt unwell. It so happens that the days I am unwell (at the office, home or wherever) are always the days I have a lot of stress. Also I KNOW it's not the chemical, because when I am unstressed and happy, many of the symptoms disappear, even though I am working/living in the same place. And anyway, I have been exposed to X for twenty years; it's never worried me before.'

How can one blame the patient? What he/she said makes sense! Alas! As any serious student of logic will tell you, commonsense is NOT always logical. And even logical thinking can be off the mark sometimes and needs to be replaced by lateral thinking.

The body is not trying to get rid of exactly the same number or types of chemicals all the time, or every day. Say your body is working flat out to rid itself of the trichoroethylene you were exposed to all night long because you hung a batch of freshly dry-cleaned clothes in your wardrobe. It may be also busy trying to get rid of an accumulation of formaldehyde outgassing from your new carpet which you inhaled while watching TV.

By the time you wake up, the camel's back has a high pile of 'straws' on it. You enter the office, someone turns on the photocopier and ten minutes later, bingo! You feel unwell. The last straw broke the camel's back. You get better later on and, by the time you get home, much of the xenobiotics have outgassed from the dry-cleaning and you don't watch television as much that night.

The following day, when someone starts up the photocopier, there is still a little room on your camel's back. Hence you don't feel a thing.

Naturally, the same thing happens if your stress levels are high enough to lower your resistance, place demands upon your body, use up energy, etc.

Let's go back for a moment to detox Phase One and its bottlenecks. When the detox process is halted at this point, some of the alcohols and aldehydes may be metabolised to epoxies. These are dangerous and highly reactive chemicals. They are suspected of playing a major role in the predisposition to cancer (mutation), allergies, immune suppression and cellular ageing.

Nutritionally, the best protection against such blockages is an ample supply of zinc, GSH, selenium, magnesium and sulphur-containing amino acids (apart from meats, and fish, sulphur can be found in eggs, cruciferous vegetables, onions and garlic).

When detox pathways don't work well, chemicals get shuffled around by the body searching for a way out. In doing this they can interfere with the detox of other chemicals so that any one particular xenobiotic, which, until then was being cleared successfully, all of a sudden starts to pile up. Much like it sometimes happens when there is an accident and the police start to divert the traffic to avoid a traffic jam, only to create another one somewhere else. How frustrating!

What can happen to your body as a result of all this?

The person who until that day was unaffected by the toluene outgassing from his/her carpet, feels unwell at home. If he/she tells anyone, chances are they will shout 'neurotic'. Unless of course, they are familiar with the biochemistry of detox.

When considering environmental illness, it is well worth keeping in mind a few simple principles:

- Many illnesses do not have a single, easily identifiable cause.
- Everyone is biochemically unique.
- In a group of sick people each individual may have his/her particular trigger or allergen that is responsible for much the same symptoms.
- The opposite is also possible. The same trigger, allergy, chemical or whatever, may provoke different symptoms, even different illnesses in different individuals.
- Any material which outgasses, which can be breathed, will enter the bloodstream and may affect any organ, including the brain — even if you can't smell it.
- Once one becomes sensitised or overloaded, chances are one will become more and more sensitive to more and more factors — be they foods, chemicals or inhalants.
- Once exposed, there occurs sometimes a resetting phenomena, whereby one becomes affected more easily by lower doses or shorter exposure times. The symptoms may become more severe with repeated exposure.
- The brain is a common target of xenobiotics.
- The environment is not constant. It changes all the time. For that reason, among others, reactions or symptoms are not always the same, as they depend both on the state of the environment at the time and the individual's capacity to detox. Reducing the total load, therefore, must be the most basic step.
- In practice, this means that even apparently minor, superficial factors that are not known to provoke noticeable symptoms or reactions must be eliminated if possible. Such factors as: allergies, moulds sensitivities, candida, dust mites, hypoglycaemia, hormonal problems, pre-menstrual tension, nutritional deficiencies, imbalances or dependencies (even excesses).

So remember:
Detox, avoid, protect and educate yourself and others.

ARE YOU CHEMICALLY OVERLOADED?

Dr Mark Donohoe, who knows more than most people about the effects of chemicals, agrees that there are some basic concepts about the diagnosis and treatment of chemical toxicity that everybody should be familiar with, so we have put together the following hints list:

Hints for suspecting chemical toxicity

- Suspect chemical problems if you have seen several doctors and still do not have a conclusive diagnosis.
- Consider the problem is chemical overload when the diagnosis that has been made proves to be wrong after a closer examination.
- The same applies if you know you are quite normal but have been told you are 'neurotic', 'hysterical' or that 'it's all in your head'.
- Note that chemical toxicity can elicit symptoms which can mimic almost any disease.
- Consider chemicals when you have been told that your problem is an overloaded liver, a congested digestive system or poor elimination due to bad eating habits, without having been told exactly WHAT caused the overloading, congestion or poor elimination.
- Always keep in mind that what are good habits for someone else could turn out to be very bad for you. Every week I see at least one unfortunate person who is allergic to grains (gluten) and became very ill only after switching to a diet very high in complex carbohydrates like bran.
- Suspect something if you live or have lived near a power station, in heavily polluted areas or places known to have been heavily contaminated, such as some of our beaches, the Ourimbah/Mangrove Mountain and Coffs Harbour regions, or if you work in an industry that uses lots of chemicals, such as farming, plastics, rubber manufacturers, etc.
- Be alert if, in spite of a good diet and supplements, you suffer with chronic or recurring infections, candida, allergies or such immune diseases as arthritis, lupus, diabetes, multiple sclerosis, cancer, thyroid problems, etc.
- Remember that even if you are found to be chemically sensitive, or overloaded with toxins, it is still possible you suffer other, concurrent health problems with different causes which may need different treatments.

- Make sure you see a diagnostician/therapist who knows how to order and interpret the special tests needed.

If you are found to suffer from chemical toxicity, overload or sensitivity, make sure your therapist explains to you the concepts of total load and unloading. In addition:

Hints for the treatment of chemical toxicity

- Exercise some form of environmental control.
- Avoid all known allergens (foods, chemicals, inhalants) to which you are sensitive.
- Arrange to have your allergies desensitised or neutralised if possible.
- Take antioxidant supplements, but make sure the type, form and composition are tailored to your individual needs.
- Start some steps towards detoxification, but beware of fasting or exercise without supervision because these could cause a crisis or worsen your condition.
- Make sure the correct tests are used to diagnose your problems, whether chemical or otherwise. Some test centres in Australia either do not have the equipment to detect low enough levels or use techniques that are outdated.

Simple ways to reduce your exposure to toxic chemicals

- Do not use fossil fuels in your home for cooking or heating (kerosene, wood, oil) and preferably no natural gas. If you do have gas cooking, have it checked for leaks and shut off the main when not in use.
- Do not have carpets in the house, especially in the bedroom. If this is not possible, have the plainest carpet available and have the formaldehyde steam cleaned out of it. This may require more than one treatment.
- Use only water-based paints and avoid veneers, oil paints or wallpaper.
- Do not use chipboard, particleboard or plywood. Especially not for shelves in your bedroom or for a bedhead.
- Do not drink tap water unless you use a filter with both a carbon filter and reverse osmosis. Otherwise use distilled water.

- Avoid long, hot showers (baths are OK). When anyone else has a hot shower, remember to shut the door and open the window. Don't allow the chlorine-loaded steam to enter the rest of the house.
- Do not wear freshly dry-cleaned clothes. Air them for a few hours and do not hang them up in your bedroom's wardrobe until they are well aired.
- Avoid self-service petrol stations and NEVER eat or drink anything sold in close proximity to one.
- Do not leave your car in the hot sun. If unavoidable, air the car well before driving away. Remember that toxic outgassing from plastic increases with temperature.
- Do not use chlorinated cleaners to wash floors or remove mould from bathrooms.
- Avoid nail polish and especially polish removers.
- Do not jog or exercise strenuously anywhere near vehicle traffic, factories or any other source of pollution.
- Remember that chemical sensitivity can occur after one single massive exposure to one chemical as well as by chronic exposure to small amounts of a number of chemicals.
- Remember the principle of *biochemical individuality*.
- Duration and intensity of exposure, one's genetic, inherited resistance, nutrition, biochemical functions, general health and emotional state will determine who is affected by what and for how long as well as how badly.

BASIC RULES
There is a general set of rules for chemical CFS sufferers or, if you prefer, environmentally ill people:

- Understand, and get your doctor to learn, that xenobiotics can take up residence within macrophages and produce no symptoms or illness until further stimulation by an antigen (allergen, virus, bacteria), causes them to begin a flood of interlukins, thus altering dramatically that individual's immune response capabilities, sometimes without measurably altering the actual numbers of immune components.
- The effects of exposure to xenobiotics has been shown to be time-synergistic. In the case of solvents, this means that if someone is exposed to TWO solvents simultaneously, the mean

time before damage occurs is reduced from twelve years (the time for a single chemical to cause damage) to about seven years. Exposure to THREE solvents can shorten this to around four years. There is a good possibility that the same or a worse degree of exponentiality occurs with many other xenobiotics.
- Remember that moulds (fungi) can be toxic as well as cause allergies. Fungi can produce their own very powerful mycotoxins.
- Pets should be kept out of the homes of allergic individuals, even if they are not actually allergic to the animal itself.
- Hang dry-cleaning in the bathroom overnight, after taking the plastic wrap off.
- Avoid self-service petrol stations and do not buy any food that has been prepared near a service station.
- No gas-, kerosene- or wood-burning appliances.
- Remove carpets from bedrooms, especially in children's rooms. Even if they are healthy, a carpeted room will increase their chances of becoming allergic.
- If the home has been treated with chemicals to control pests, do not vacuum clean too often. You'll only re-distribute some of the dried up chemicals into the air. Have the carpet thoroughly cleaned, without using more chemicals, first.
- Avoid long, very hot showers and, if anyone is having one, keep the bathroom door shut and the window open.
- Avoid nail polishes and removers.
- Never sleep in a freshly painted or wallpapered room.
- Switch electric blankets off at the main plug site before getting into bed.
- Do not have a clock radio near the bedhead.
- Do not have a bedroom over your garage.
- If you are allergic, and especially if you are asthmatic, avoid BBQs and charcoal-cooked foods.
- Avoid permanent press clothes and do not sleep on synthetic mattresses or polyester sheets.
- Use natural, non-toxic paints and do not use wood oils and oil paints in the bedroom.
- If you want to nurture your liver, sleep between 8 p.m. and 11 p.m. as this is the most important recuperative time for that organ.

- Avoid jogging or riding a bicycle in a metropolitan area and NEVER do it where there is vehicle traffic.
- Use only filtered or distilled water.
- Boiling of water can be dangerous, especially for small children. All you will achieve is to further concentrate any dangerous chemicals present.

If chemicals are a problem and if they are part of your CFS, either as a cause or as an effect, you will have to detox:

- *your diet:* eat as naturally as possible; check food allergies/intolerances and make sure the diet is optimal FOR YOU
- *your body:* avoid drugs whenever possible, including alcohol; use as few chemicals on your body as possible; use hypoallergenic natural products whenever possible
- *your home/bedroom:* clean up dust, dust mites, mould, outgassing sources, etc.; use plants to soak up chemicals (see What You Can Do to Help Yourself p. 132 later in this section); obtain advice from experts in different areas, such as water filters, air-conditioning, de-humidifiers, anti-mould and anti-dust mite procedures; be careful, as there are some firms around advertising such services that will take your money, and not do a suitable job; ring one of the environmental groups to find who is recommended and who is not by the experts and
- *your mind:* remember that bad, angry, negative thinking is stressful; love and laughter are the best medicine.

CHECKLIST
In general, if you suffer with an environmental illness, and are not improving despite treatment, here is a program to remind you what can, and should, be done. Ask yourself and your therapist the following:

- Has your doctor evaluated the threat posed by the mould in your bedroom and other parts of the house you spend a lot of time in and have your arranged for removal, control and desensitisation or neutralisation, as needed?
- Have you ruled out food allergies and intolerance?
- Have you checked for and treated candida?

- Is your diet as free of additives, chemicals, colourings, preservatives, etc., as possible?
- Have you taken the necessary supplements/medications as directed?
- Is your mind in a healing mode?

Neurotoxins

Anything that affects our nervous system is likely to affect our immune system as well. And it often works the other way around. If something disrupts our immunity, chances are that our nervous system (brain, etc.) will be disturbed too. And that is probably the main physiological reason why we all experience mood disturbances when we are sick. You know what I mean. You have a cold, a sore throat and become grumpy, irritable.

With many, if not all illnesses, in fact, one is likely to experience some mood problems. Some very physical illnesses involving immunity (lupus for instance) provoke mood disorders or psychiatric disturbances as the FIRST signs and symptoms. And I don't have to tell you that CFS sufferers experience all sorts of emotional, mood, psychological or psychiatric problems.

Some, like depression, may well be a result of the fact that one tends to be depressed when illness persists. No one likes to be sick. In many cases, however, the depression, or anxiety or whatever may well be an integral part of CFS; one of the symptoms in the cluster of symptoms that characterise this syndrome. It can even be the major one.

There is little doubt in the minds of most scientists involved in the treatment of CFS, and in the search for its causes and effects, that this syndrome involves both the nervous system *and* the immune system, especially since we know that they and their functions are closely associated with one another.

The brain is, of course, part of what we call the 'central nervous system' and disturbances of that system can give rise to physical, neurological and mental symptoms and illnesses ranging from peripheral neuropathy to schizophrenia. That neuropsychiatric and neurophysiological symptoms should be so abundant in patients suffering from CFS should not surprise us at all.

The diagnosis of human illness is, in many ways, an exercise in the detection of biochemical and/or physiological disturbances in the body. People only become aware of the effects of such disturbances if they happen to cause what we call 'symptoms' and they are the body's own warning signals that something is amiss.

We can become ill for many different reasons: trauma, malignant cells, infectious agents (viruses, bacteria, fungi, etc.) or simply because we do not receive sufficient nutrients to enable our body to ward off an attack. Whatever the causes, symptoms can vary greatly from person to person and from illness to illness. Of course the symptoms one actually 'feels' can have their origin in different parts of the body.

And therein lies one of the great problems of 'modern medicine'. We tend to think of body functions only in terms of the organs responsible for them, almost as if these organs existed as independent, self-contained units. But, in fact, each organ is totally dependent on every other organ. For example, it is pointless to talk about heart disease as if the heart existed in total isolation. Its own blood supply depends on a healthy circulation, which in turn depends on nutrients — from the foods we eat, the gases we breathe and the fluids we drink. To some extent, our circulation is also dependent on our physical activity which, in turn, can be affected by anything from our sex life to our working conditions.

Then there are our brain functions, which are largely regulated by the hormones the brain produces from amino acids present in the food we eat. The brain cannot obtain these unless the foods are first digested and then absorbed.

However, the brain is a very delicate organ and its intricate hormonal system can be unbalanced, its synchronicity thrown out of kilter and its regulatory neurotransmitter chemicals antagonised, deactivated or inhibited by a considerable number of substances, natural or otherwise.

Alcohol and cannabis have well-known effects on the brain. What is not so well known is that there is a particular class of chemicals whose effects are very subtle but treacherous — often at very small doses. These are the neurotoxins; substances which can damage the nervous system and which can therefore cause almost any emotional or behavioural symptom — from hallucinations to depression, from sleeplessness to dementia and from memory loss to psychosis. Inevitably, they affect the immune system.

Changes brought about by the neurotoxins are very often such that most people affected have no idea what is causing their symptoms. That is bad enough. Often, however, their doctors are equally unaware of the real cause of the problem and may begin a long search for a physical cause for each of the symptoms; the early warnings of neurotoxicity can be quite subtle and misleading.

Tingling and numbness of the fingers or toes, slight tremors or just feeling 'shaky', slight unco-ordination, impotence and decreased sensations of touch are all characteristic physical symptoms. Later, perhaps years after the initial exposure, there may be some general pains, problems with vision, a decreased sense of smell and taste, lowered alertness, loss of memory, lethargy, irritability and eventually depression, hallucinations and psychosis — or a combination of these.

Many of these effects are irreversible because the central nervous system often cannot repair or replace some of the damaged or lost cells. The consequences on the human intellect are therefore profound and long lasting, if not permanent. Because of the nature of the presenting symptoms, these are often attributed to an excessive workload, advancing age or even the ubiquitous 'stress'.

One additional problem of neurotoxicity is that because it almost invariably involves some degree of impairment of an individual's faculty of judgement, neurotoxins may be responsible for a great number of industrial accidents.

A word of warning: bear in mind that the 'official' disclaimer about this or that poisonous chemical additive, in which the 'authority' claims that a certain chemical is absolutely harmless in the permitted quantities, can be misleading. These amounts, usually measured in parts per million, are pronounced safe for human consumption after a number of hapless laboratory animals have been given beverages laced with the particular toxins in increasing amounts until the lethal or carcinogenic dose has been established. No attempt is made to measure the synergistic effects of multiple additives.

TOXINS AND THE ENVIRONMENT

Traditional definitions of toxicology for the most part encompass damage to the various body tissues and the likelihood of death. In the past few years, however, we have seen a shift in emphasis, which has resulted in more focus on environmental issues and concern with the consequences of long-term exposure to low levels of chemicals. Many scientific investigators, including myself, feel that one of the primary criteria that should be investigated is that of 'functions'.

Since function defines life, and since many toxic substances disrupt the smooth functioning of a body, the effects of exposure to toxins should be studied by examining changes in various functions brought about by that exposure. Behavioural toxicology is, in fact, a measurement of subtle functional disorders.

Within such a framework of reference, lead poisoning can be seen as a major hazard to behavioural and mental health. An American report on lead by the National Research Council, which describes the medical and biological effects of environmental pollutants (Select Committee on Nutrition and Human Needs, June 1977), made the following statement:

> The early symptoms of lead poisoning are subtle, subjective and nonspecific and therefore not so readily recognised in children ... In children such mild symptoms are often overlooked or attributed to other disease states, so that poisoning due to lead is more likely to be recognised first at a late or severe stage on the basis of nervous system involvement (acute encephalopathy).

Another example is that of a Brethism, a syndrome of mercury intoxication, characterised by a cluster of symptoms that mimics the behaviour of a tormented neurotic.

> I got a sore mouth, had dizzy spells, and began to be so weak and tired that at night when I got home from work it was hard to even get my supper and do my work. I got so grouchy and nervous I would cry at nothing ... I often wake suddenly and have a fluttering feeling like I was scared and floating

in space. I kept feeling worse and getting trembly and nervous, and my eyes were bloodshot. I seemed to forget things so easily.

This statement is not from a 'neurotic' but from a woman who was constantly exposed to mercury in an electric motor components factory. Such symptoms remind us that human behaviour reflects the conditions of the whole human organism, not just the liver, heart, brain, or an enzyme system. As the study of neurotoxins makes clear, it is the whole organism that complains of pains, becomes confused, irritable or depressed. Hopefully further medical research will be addressed to the study of synergism and the less obvious causes of disease.

ETHOXYETHANOL
This is a widely used industrial solvent related to the alcohol found in lacquers, dyes, varnish removers and many other industrial processes. It has always been regarded as 'safe'; when the compound was extensively tested in laboratory animals it was shown to produce no toxic effects. Even pregnant rats did not suffer when exposed to doses equivalent to half the allowable limits. But their offspring did. Subsequent tests showed significant changes in brain chemistry and after-birth behaviour.

B. K. Nelson, a scientist at the National Institute for Occupational Safety and Health (USA), carried out another test. He gave some pregnant rats enough ethoxyethanol to be safe for them but toxic to their offspring. At the same time he mixed a little alcohol into their drinking water. The effects of this combination on the brain neurochemistry of the offspring were twice as severe as those caused by ethoxyethanol alone.

The implications of this are frightening. It is quite possible that a great many people who are infrequently exposed to small amounts of ethoxyethanol may suffer no symptoms — at least no observable ones — from such exposure. If the same people consume regular amounts of alcohol, the toxicity of ethoxyethanol is potentiated, so that their children may suffer serious neurological consequences.

CARBON DISULPHIDE
Discovered in the latter part of the eighteenth century, carbon disulphide was originally used as a general anaesthetic. A Scottish

surgeon, I. Simpson, reported in 1840 that he was no longer using it because it caused hallucinations, headaches and nausea in his patients. Within a few years carbon disulphide began to be used extensively as a solvent in industrial processes. Soon, it was discovered that carbon disulphide could 'soften' rubber at any temperature, thus making possible the many modern uses for this product. Such things as raincoats, rubber toys and balloons became easier to manufacture because of the properties which it imparted to an otherwise hard rubber. Of course, anyone working with this substance was exposed to its deadly vapours.

Alan Anderson, writing in *Psychology Today,* tells us that in 1902 a British publication, *Dangerous Trades,* described a factory in which the windows were barred to prevent crazed workers from leaping forth during their delirious attacks.

Meanwhile the rubber industry has developed, causing untold thousands of unsuspecting workers to lose their health and sanity. Nothing was done about it, and it is still causing problems today. In Finland, workers in modern, well-ventilated and clean rayon factories, which use carbon disulphide in their processes, have been tested and shown to have lost some neuromuscular speed, working capacity, intelligence and psychomotor ability.

NITRATES

Although nitrates themselves are not particularly toxic, when they change to nitrites or nitrosamines they become quite dangerous. This can happen during the digestive process. They are suspected of being carcinogenic but a lesser known and just as frightening capacity of nitrites is that of causing methemoglobimia — a condition in which blood no longer carries an adequate amount of oxygen. A small child thus affected may turn blue and suffer permanent brain damage as a result. As it grows up, the child's impairment may show in several ways. Thus, nitrates can indirectly become neurotoxic.

One way in which this can happen is by feeding babies with formulae made up with well water that has a high content of nitrites. Well water can easily become contaminated by pesticides and other chemicals which are used in agriculture. Sometimes animal wastes can be high in nitrate content and this may affect local water supplies. Methemoglobimia can also be caused by air polluted with vanadium.

VOLATILE FUELS

According to some studies workers exposed to jet fuels have poor scores in behavioural tests that demand a high degree of concentration. Statistically, such workers were found to have more psychiatric illnesses and symptoms of depression and neurotic behaviour.

Similar results were obtained in studies of people exposed to paint solvents. A Scandinavian study reported in *Psychology Today* (July 1982) revealed that when fifty-two house painters were studied they scored lower than control on tests of intellectual capacity, psychomotor co-ordination, memory and reaction time. Totally oblivious of the danger, the workers sometimes washed their hands in methyl-n-butyl ketone, a powerful neurotoxin capable of severely damaging the central nervous system.

Similarly, surgeons and other operating theatre personnel are often exposed to anaesthetic gases which can escape from pressure-relief valves used during operations. Nitrous oxides and halothane, when inhaled in concentrations as low as 50 parts per million and 1 part per million respectively, can affect recent memory, visual perception acuity and cognitive motor responses — the very skills needed in an operating theatre.

ALUMINIUM

This metal has been implicated in many neurological problems, especially Alzheimer's disease. Antacids, deodorants and some medications are the most common sources but some researchers claim that cooking with aluminium cookware may create problems. Others disclaim this. Be that as it may, aluminium cookware and fluoridated water may be a dangerous combination.

MERCURY

Quicksilver, as mercury used to be known, has always been regarded as somewhat magical, as well as sinister, because of its unique property — it is the only metal to be liquid at room temperature. Its toxic properties have been well known since mediaeval times and it was used extensively as a poison for both suicide and murder. Strangely enough, mercury was also probably the first metal compound to be employed therapeutically.

The effects of mercury poisoning are horrendous and difficult to diagnose. One of the problems is that the appearance of neurological damage is taken as the standard to be used when allowing for daily intake or exposure. However, some damage may occur before overt symptoms manifest themselves.

Sources of mercury include some bleaches and cosmetics, certain medications, some lenses-cleaning solutions, dental amalgam, industrial photography ingredients, mirrors, tattoos, batteries, some electrical equipment, thermometers and some alloys such as tin, copper or nickel which may have mercury in them.

Recently there has been a great deal of furore over the possibility that CFS may be caused by dental mercury. I believe that in some cases this is so. If, after eliminating other possibilities, patients with lots of fillings or with a history of onset of illness occurring shortly after amalgam replacement fail to improve, we arrange for our dental associate (who by the way is a member of the natural health society) to investigate and, if needed, remove and replace suspect fillings. I must say that I have seen cases where nothing helped until this was done. In some, the improvement was miraculous. Many have side-effects at first, then improve slowly in a few months.

Mercury and vegetarians

One of the ways the body eliminates mercury is by combining it with sulphur-containing amino acids and then eliminating the product.

The principal sources of methionine, one of the main sulphur amino acids, are eggs, meats, fish, poultry and dairy foods. Diets high in methionine, and other sulphur amino acids which are often made from methionine, afford some protection against mercury poisoning, but place a great strain on the body reserves of vitamin B6, which should always be taken as an additional supplement with such a diet. Vegetarian diets, especially vegan ones, are likely to be low in sulphur amino acids. Therefore, the people most at risk from the effect of mercury poisoning are vegetarians.

Mercury also causes a reduction in vitamin C levels within the brain. One of the principal reasons for the therapeutic use of vitamin C in treating heavy metal intoxication is the ability of this vitamin to form complexes with metals which are then 'chelated' out of the body via urinary excretion. One has to bear in mind that the brain has a high capacity for ascorbic acid retention and it is possible that this property may extend to ascorbate complexes. Pectin, found in apples, and vitamin E appear to be the safest supplements available for protection, coupled with a diet high in methionine and vitamin B6.

Mercury and cholesterol

In the 1990s ageing humans perceive the flutter of death's wing, and inevitably start to worry about their hearts. And that means their cholesterol levels. Pride in one's golfing handicap is often replaced by boasting about cholesterol levels. Inevitably, the high cholesterol individual looks for ways to lower cholesterol levels. According to the renowned cardiologist, Michael Oliver, of Edinburgh, Scotland, lowering cholesterol levels may pose a serious health risk for some individuals.

It looks like a sudden rise in cholesterol levels, in spite of a reasonable diet, may be one of nature's ways to protect us from mercury poisoning. If one is exposed to excessive mercury, perhaps because of amalgam dental fillings, the body will try to get rid of it with cholesterol.

A sudden lowering of its levels can cause mercury to shift towards nerve and brain cells causing symptoms such as depression, irritability, neuromuscular and immune problems. According to new research results, the primary target organs for mercury appear to be the thyroid and pituitary glands (in that order), then brain, liver and kidneys. A recently published book *Chronic Mercury Toxicity,* by Harold Queen claims that whenever there is a suspicion of mercury toxicity, one should not enter into a cholesterol-lowering program without first undergoing a series of intravenous ascorbate (vitamin C) procedures for detoxification.

In my experience, with many cases of suspected mercury contribution to CFS I have found that the chances of amalgam replacement helping the CFS condition without causing the transient side-effects often associated with that procedure are greatly enhanced by undergoing first a series of IVC infusions.

Mercury and candida

Because candida infections are such a common part of CFS and because I have often found that until the candida infection has been treated successfully CFS may not respond to treatment, it is worth reading what Dr Alfred V. Zamm has to say about yet another weapon in the fight against systemic yeast infection (candidiasis). According to the author, mercury in dental fillings can adversely affect our immune resistance to the point where treatment for candida can fail unless the fillings are first removed.

Neither chelation nor vitamin C therapy alone are able to reduce mercury poisoning. Selenium, however, binds mercury and, according to Dr Zamm, renders it biologically inactive. Garlic contains selenium. Taking large amounts of garlic may, therefore, work in three ways in the fight against candida: (1) it acts as a general antibiotic with anti-candida properties; (2) it helps to restore a balanced gut flora; and (3) it will help the body's immune system to recover its strength. Care must be taken, however, not to begin garlic treatment too soon, because the nutrient may drive some of the candida into the deeper recesses of the villi, in the gut, making them less amenable to destruction. To help avoid this condition, taking the proper medications together with essential fatty acids (preferably in micelle-liquid form), will potentiate the effects of nystatin. Also helpful is an acid stomach, hence hydrochloric acid supplements are indicated while antacids (alkalisers) should be avoided during therapy.

There is, of course, a great deal of controversy over dental mercury and its possible effects on human health. The official stance of the Australian Dental Association is that amalgams are safe, yet the evidence suggesting otherwise is considerable. Medical scientists have been able to cause remarkable immune alterations by introducing relatively small amounts of mercury in humans.

No discussion on mercury would be complete without mentioning the champion of them all, world-renowned dentist, Hal Huggins. Dr Huggins has carefully explained the dangers of modern dentistry. He says:

> Methyl mercury is 100 times more toxic than elemental mercury and the literature is rich in describing many mechanisms of methylation within the human body. Bacteria in the mouth, stomach, small intestine, large intestine (several hundred species) are capable of methylation. Even intestinal yeast (fungi) and mucosal cells can change elemental mercury into methyl mercury.

SELENIUM

Selenium combines with mercury, so a diet adequate in selenium-containing foods and drinking water with some selenium helps to protect against mercury poisoning.

Selenium itself can be highly poisonous so dietary supplements in very large doses should be taken only under medical supervision. Selenium is, nevertheless, a very important and essential mineral. People who drink water with low selenium content, or who otherwise become selenium deficient, have been found to be prone to cardiovascular diseases. Several reports have also linked cancer with a selenium-deficient diet, but an excess intake is just as bad and in this case far worse than taking in too little.

We know that selenium can pollute water in areas where selenium-rich soil is irrigated. When animals eat the plants that grow there, the metal damages the foetus and can cause the birth of deformed offspring.

MANGANESE

This is another potentially toxic metal. It is added to jet fuel to make the outpouring smoke less black — reducing the size of airborne particles so that they tend to disperse without being quite so visible. The particles, however, can penetrate lung tissues and cause serious respiratory and neurological damage. Manganese is also used in ordinary petrol, as a replacement for lead, which is unwise as it is probably just as harmful.

A brochure distributed by a leading hair analysis centre in the United States described the symptoms of manganese toxicity as very similar, if not indistinguishable from, those of schizophrenia, and adds that 'symptomatic deficiency of manganese has not been demonstrated in humans'.

However, manganese is useful in combination with some other vitamins to counteract side-effects of the phenothiazine drugs.

Manganese seems to be a potentially toxic substance that can, nevertheless, be used effectively in the treatment of several diseases. It has been used extensively in orthomolecular psychiatry but, as I have pointed out, its widespread use as a supplement in high doses is potentially dangerous to some people unless administered and taken under supervision.

TRICHLOROETHANE

This rather frightening sounding chemical may sound remote but it is, in fact, a common thinner used in products like liquid paper. It is one of the milder chlorinated hydrocarbons which act as a thinner by keeping particles light and easily spread. Hydrocarbons and fluorocarbons can, if inhaled in large enough quantities, cause symptoms similar to those which follow alcohol intoxication. They also cause headaches, ringing in the ears and hallucinations not unlike those triggered by LSD. If enough hydrocarbons are inhaled, convulsions and eventually a state of coma may be the unhappy results.

Many people are unwittingly exposed to hydrocarbon and fluorocarbon fumes. Sensitive individuals, especially children, can suffer from twitching muscles and hyperactive reflexes as a result. Those who are hypersensitive or allergic to these compounds may also suffer extreme behavioural disorders because of exposure.

People, particularly teenagers, sometimes abuse this substance, seeking a euphoric 'high'.

POLLUTION, CHEMICALS, ADDITIVES AND THEIR EFFECTS

There is little doubt now that xenobiotics can cause or aggravate CFS. One of the problems is that, when they do not seem to do so in an overt manner, people tend to dismiss the possibility.

Because of the capacity of chemicals to elicit neurological and psychiatric symptoms, and because such symptoms are an integral part of the CFS picture, we should be familiar with some of the possible effects.

Arsenic: Giddiness, headaches, general weakness, fatigue.
Boron: Restlessness, unco-ordination, aggressiveness, jitteriness, disorientation.
Cadmium: Fatigue, lack of taste or smell dysfunctions, increased heart disease risk.
Copper: Irritability, poor concentration span, hyperactivity.
Manganese: Psychiatric symptoms (French miners exposed to it showed symptoms indistinguishable from schizophrenia).
Mercury: Tremors, lack of co-ordination, speech problems, psychiatric problems.
Nickel: Headaches, insomnia, delirium, irritability.

Selenium: Dizziness, lassitude, depression, fatigue.
Tin: Limb weaknesses, vertigo, photophobia.
Pesticides: Neurological, metabolic and psychiatric disturbances.
Chlorine: Q fever in livestock (can be transferred to humans).
Nitrates: Possibly cancers.

This list contains only 10 per cent of the total possible contaminants. Of course, we have many different forms of pollution: noise, asbestos, cadmium, aerosols, propellants, DDT, dioxin, 245T, fluoride, carbon dioxide, industrial solvents, detergents, chlorine, fluorocarbons, colourings … the list is endless, and so are the symptoms, the problems and the long-term side-effects caused by them.

It has been said, with some justification, that almost any substance can provoke a reaction in a susceptible individual. That is to say, humans can be or become allergic or hypersensitive to almost anything.

We now have serious reason to believe that the higher the load of pollutants — chemical, biochemical, environmental, emotional (stress) — the more likely an exposed individual is to become allergic to the substance or to a number of environmental agents to which he may be exposed at a moment of lowered resistance.

Other studies have shown that a deficiency in a single vitamin or mineral (or multiple deficiencies) increased the allergic response of the individual exposed to the allergen and increased the toxic effects of pollutants.

WHAT CAN WE DO ABOUT THIS?

There are many other effects of pollution which can be eliminated, avoided or, at least, counter-balanced, by sensible approaches and proper nutrition. Let me give you some examples.

Everybody (especially pregnant women and breast-feeding mothers) should try to avoid using pesticides in the home. Pests can be eliminated, or at least minimised, by the judicious use of herbs. Cat thyme, for example, is what one would call a 'broad spectrum' insect repellant. Crushed leaves of pennyroyal will help to keep mosquitos away from your child, and tansy will tend to repel flies.

Vitamin C supplements will help neutralise the effects of nitrates in foods by blocking the formation of potentially carcinogenic nitrosamines. The slow release of this vitamin will afford some degree of protection from meal to meal and from snacks taken during the day.

Ozone and nitrogen dioxide, common pollutants in Western cities, increase the degeneration of lipid components of lung cells and the subsequent formation of free radicals (these are toxic particles, formed during certain chemical reactions in the body, which are thought to be responsible for ageing, cancer and degenerative diseases).

Poor nutrition in general tends to create a vacuum that allows heavy metals like cadmium and lead to accumulate in the body.

Vitamin C and zinc are both known to inhibit the absorption of lead, and to help the body dispose of it. A lack of calcium and/or vitamin D3 predisposes an individual (especially a child) to bronchial constriction, which causes breathing difficulties such as asthma. These deficiencies have such an effect on health that they may cause mental performance to decline rapidly.

Allergy, which is aggravated by pollution and by vitamin and mineral deficiencies, is a significant factor in a child's learning ability. Allergy can indirectly affect a child's learning ability by causing poor health; asthma, sinusitis and hay fever are examples of this. In other cases the brain is the target for the allergy (which is then termed neuro-allergy or brain allergy), and the reaction almost invariably includes decreased performance at school and behavioural problems ranging from total lethargy to hyperactivity and aggressiveness.

HOW TO HELP YOUR BODY TO ELIMINATE TOXIC HEAVY METALS AND CHEMICALS

- Pacific brown kelp contains algin, a substance known to prevent absorption of some toxic metals.
- Apples contain pectin, which produces substances known to attach themselves to heavy metals thus preventing their absorption.
- Calcium is absorbed preferentially to some heavy metals, especially lead.

- Vitamin C, vitamin A, beta carotene, vitamin E, methionine, L-cysteine, L-lysine and taurine are available either as natural amino acids in some protein foods like fish and eggs or in onions, garlic, beans and legumes, or they can be bought as supplements. These are all helpful detoxing agents.
- Chelation is useful only in some cases. Calcium disodium EDT acetate chelates mainly zinc, copper, cadmium, manganese and nickel. It has little effect on mercury, arsenic and gold. Disodium EDT acetate chelates calcium. Dimercapol chelates arsenic, mercury and gold. Penicillamine (cuprimine) chelates copper, iron and lead.
- Selenium protects against mercury poisoning.
- Zinc helps to counteract some of the effects of lead, cadmium and mercury.

Pesticides

A patient of mine, Vicky, visited her parents one Mother's Day. Within 10 minutes of entering their house she started to feel ill. By the time 30 minutes had elapsed, Vicky felt dizzy, nauseous and had to lie down. She was taken back to her own flat where she went straight to bed and remained there, almost incapacitated, for five days. Vicky suffers from many allergies, is chemically overloaded and is also extremely sensitive to chemicals in general and pesticides in particular. Her father had his house debugged by a pest control firm just a few days before Mother's Day. The week after Mother's Day, Vicky's father decided that, since his daughter could not be exposed again to the pesticide residues still lingering on in his house, he would go to her. Which is exactly what he did the following weekend. As soon as he embraced his daughter, she started to feel dizzy and had to lie down again. This time it took her only two days to recover. Infinitesimal amounts of pesticides still embedded in his jacket caused the reaction.

How, you might ask, can anyone be so sensitive? After all, millions of people have their homes sprayed regularly and the use of pesticides is very common. Surely there must be something else wrong with her? Yes, there is something else wrong with

Vicky. The something else, however, is nothing more sinister than a predisposition to allergies and a susceptibility to chemicals. Both are common problems. They are more likely to occur if someone else in your family is, or was, atopic (allergic) and suffers, or has suffered, attacks of sinusitis, asthma, hay fever, hives, dermatitis and other allergic diseases. In Vicky's case it is just a matter of degree.

Some of you may have heard of a scientist called Dr Roger Williams, who first expounded the principles of Biochemical Individuality some 40 odd years ago. That principle is the cornerstone of orthomolecular and nutritional medicine. After all, we can easily understand that if our climate became progressively colder, we would need more and more protective clothing to keep warm, to function normally. In our increasingly polluted world we may well need more and more nutrients to keep us healthy by antagonising at least some of the effects of man-made chemicals. From time to time every health practitioner sees individuals who may need many thousands of milligrams of Vitamin C each day (far in excess of the inadequate official RDA) just to survive in our hostile world. The same applies, of course, to most vitamins, minerals, amino acids and foods.

The irony of it all is that many, if not most of the protective enzymes reside in the liver and this organ is the first to suffer from the effects of chemicals. This can render the liver progressively less efficient at clearing the very chemicals which make it inefficient in the first place.

If you are unlucky enough to be born with a genetic susceptibility to liver damage, as well as a slow chemical clearance rate, the odds are stacked against you. If you are chronically exposed to low levels of chemicals, this will tend to make you allergic. If you are *already* allergic, this exposure will either 'unmask' the allergy or, if the allergy is already overt, make it worse. As James Scheer, editor of *Let's Live* once said, 'Everybody is at least potentially allergic [hypersensitive] to something — and there are thousands upon thousands of "somethings" around.'

Recent studies at the Environmental Health Center at Dallas, USA, have substantiated the numerous animal studies which have shown serious consequences of chronic low-level chemical

exposure. Which individual, and how they are affected, depends upon:
- The amounts and biological activity of the chemical.
- The length of exposure.
- The state of an individual's health in general and his particular biochemical status, stress load and psychological (mental) health.
- Genetic (heriditary) influences.
- Biochemical individuality.
- Age, sex, cultural and ethnic background.

Depending on these factors, one or more body systems may be affected. After all, a chain is only as strong as its weakest link — and that is the first to break. Often a combination of systems are affected. It is not uncommon to see a patient with pre-menstrual tension, poor digestion and chronic sinusitis, all due to extreme sensitivity to low-grade but chronic exposure to nothing more sinister than the dye in one's carpet! The problem is that chemical toxicity often mimics other diseases and is sometimes mistaken for signs of an individual system, or organ, sickness. Thus people with a cluster of unexplainable symptoms are often referred to a psychiatrist when an examination of the specific organ system cannot reveal a pathological abnormality.

As Chinese philosophers explained thousands of years ago, macro- and microcosms reflect each other. Every day I see the clinical effects of these factors in some of my patients, yet it must be remembered that even mundane pollutants which people may come in contact with every day of their lives can damage their health.

Judith West, Senior Pharmacist in the Royal Alexandra Hospital for Children, heads the Poisons Information Centre with a group of nine other experienced pharmacists. Each of them handles more than 100 calls each and every day from parents and doctors seeking advice on chemical poisoning. Pesticides, and all of them are potentially dangerous, accounted for 2796 calls to the centre in 1988, according to Paola Totaro, Consumer Affairs Correspondent for the *Daily Telegraph* (Sydney), who interviewed Ms West in May 1989.

Simple, commonly used pesticides can contain deadly substances such as antimony, a heavy metal which corrodes and causes cellular poisoning and kidney failure. Especially dangerous are many garden sprays; even your dog's flea repellant is poisonous. In 1977, a child died after ingesting a common flea-rinse.

The term 'pesticides' covers a range of agents, including insecticides, fungicides, herbicides, fumigants and rodenticides. The modern insecticides belong to several families: organophosphates, chlorinated hydrocarbons, cabramates, botanicals, insect hormones, chemical sterilants and insect viruses.

Organophosphates are dangerous because they tend to attack a vital enzyme called acetylcholinesterase. Interference with this enzyme causes muscle and central nervous system disorders. Diarrhoea, muscular weakness, dizziness, impaired vision and shortness of breath are the more common symptoms. The danger of poisoning by pesticides increases in an inverse proportion to the amounts of sulphur-containing proteins in one's diet. Captan, for example, is a fungicide used in some cultivation and home gardening. It is almost harmless to a well-nourished person but can become deadly in a protein-deficient individual.

Although the consumption of high-fibre foods is generally recommended, and is normally beneficial to health, one must remember that excessive fibre can cause some proteins to be malabsorbed. If this happens while the person is on a low-protein diet, exposure to pesticides can be fatal. This is an important factor that should be borne in mind when a vegetarian buys a farm for his own use. Another point worth remembering, especially by those naturopaths who practise extensive fasting therapy, is that most pesticides, especially chlorinated hydrocarbons, accumulate in body fats. During prolonged fasting, these fat stores are broken down for energy, and pesticides, especially DDT, can infiltrate the blood, producing concentrations high enough to become dangerous.

The type of protein that protects against pesticides poisoning is crucial. Laboratory animals raised on soya proteins, which have a low content of methionine, experience stunted growth and liver damage if exposed to DDT. Low sulphur diets (methionine is a sulphur amino acid) cause a deficiency of vitamin A by affecting liver reserves. Cysteine is another amino acid which is said to afford some protection from pesticides. And so are most antioxidants (vitamin C, vitamin E, beta carotene and selenium).

So you throw away all the chemicals and stock up on vinegar, pyrethrum-based insect sprays, natural garlic concoctions and various eucalyptus brews. You check all the possible alternatives, become environmentally aware, read all the labels carefully so you and your family are protected until death do you part. Right? Wrong!

'Inert' ingredients are sometimes included in commercial pesticides and their effects can be worse than the active ingredients. Two such ingredients, carbon tetrachloride and chloroform, are powerful liver and central nervous system toxins. In addition, exposure to inert ingredients may facilitate the absorption, and therefore the potential toxicity, of an active ingredient so that, in spite of the active ingredients being present in 'safe' amounts, the co-existence of an inert ingredient may make that level dangerous. Confusing? You bet! And because they are used as 'inert' ingredients no warning on the labels is needed.

One must also remember that because the exact mechanism of human toxicity is completely known for only a few pesticides, authorities are reluctant to issue warnings. Due to the widespread use of pesticides, low level, but chronic, exposure to several toxic compounds in commercially grown foods and buildings that have been treated with pesticides is common. So is the leakage of such toxins into the water supplies. Please note that there are drinking water standards for only a handful of pesticides and chemicals.

The 'safe' levels for pesticides in foods are based on arbitrary statistical factors which do not take into account individual susceptibilities and, what is even worse, the potential synergistic effect of the combination of more than one chemical. Always remember that when you read an official proclamation on the 'safe' amounts of a given substance, that figure is given for that one ingredient. No allowance whatsoever is made for any possible additive effect. So you are beginning to see that even if you forgo any and all chemicals you may still be exposed to the residue of some of them in the water you drink, the food you eat and, in some cases, the air you breathe.

If you have children it is a safe bet that you want them to eat plenty of fresh fruit and vegetables. Apples, peaches, apricots, pears and many vegetables are regularly sprayed with daminozide, a pesticide accused of causing cancer. Children weigh less than adults and eat more fruit and vegetables than grown-ups. They are also biochemically more sensitive and potentially at least more easily affected. Some cancers may take decades to develop. Is your child safe?

Chemical tests at Coffs Harbour in 1987 found: DDT in milk, fish, cheese, bananas, avocados; dieldrin in milk, cheese, fish, celery, pumpkin; fenitrothion in bread, flour, cereals; endosulfan in tomatoes, lettuce beans, zucchini; carbaryl in bread, flour, cereals, bran, rice; bioresmethrin in rice and bread; chlorpyrifos-methyl in bread and cereals *(Sydney Morning Herald,* 5 September 1988).

Another report in the *Sydney Morning Herald* (5 September 1988) told of a man who 'was twitching violently and frothing at the mouth and nose when his sister found him lying on the ground ...[He] was dead on arrival at ... hospital. [He] died of methomyl poisoning. Methomyl is the active ingredient of lannate, a pesticide used extensively on fruit and vegetable crops in eastern Australia...'

Washing fruit and vegetables under the tap will not remove much of the pesticides. The only way I know is to bathe them in borax, then scrub them vigorously. This is said to at least partially reduce the concentration of chemicals on the surface of contaminated products.

So what else can we do about it? Apart from lobbying the government to ban toxic chemicals, you can buy organically grown food from reputable suppliers. Eat only free range eggs and meats from animals that have not been contaminated, are not fed hormones and roam wild, feeding on grass and soil free from pesticides and herbicides. If enough of us use only such products, suppliers will be forced to change their ways.

The SYMPTOMS of pesticide poisoning can mimic almost any illness you can think of but the most common are gastric or respiratory distress, skin problems, nervous irritability, depression and tiredness.

To detoxify yourself, if you suspect you are a victim, you should NOT, under any circumstances try to diagnose or treat yourself, as your symptoms may have other, possibly lethal causes and some seemingly sensible treatments may aggravate matters. Fasting, for example, can actually worsen the situation. So you should seek the advice of a competent health practitioner who is experienced in clinical ecology.

Some of the simple measures one may take, under supervision and guidance of a professional are: aerobic exercise, dry sauna baths, niacin flush (using niacin or nicotinic acid, a form of vitamin B3), intravenous vitamin C and a diet high in sulphur amino acids, with appropriate supplementation for enhanced liver functions.

ALTERNATIVES TO PESTICIDES

All it takes is a quick look at the many articles written on the subject and one can obtain information on the simple, natural alternatives available.

Dr Kate Short, an expert and director of the Toxic and Hazardous Chemicals Committee in Sydney, NSW, has kindly supplied me with much of the information on pesticides in this section. Dr Short is also the author of *The A-Z of Chemicals in the Home,* a book I wholeheartedly recommend to you.

What You Can Do to Help Yourself

Your home or workplace

Urea foam formaldehyde insulation (UFFI) outgasses. It emits airborne particles as it decomposes, as most plastics do. Anything that can be breathed may eventually enter the brain. According to Dr Sherry Rogers, these are some of the common symptoms of UFFI exposure: depression; fatigue; poor memory; inability to concentrate; foggy brain; headaches; dizziness; spacy feelings; facial flushing; burning eyes/throat; laryngitis; chronic cough; asthma; arthritis; skin rashes; heart palpitations.

I could fill a book with list after list of common sources of chemicals such as formaldehyde. It would make boring reading.

Much more interesting for you is to learn that there are all sorts of things you can do to minimise and sometimes counteract exposure effects. One thing you can do is test your house (which, we have seen, is far from being a restful retreat and can even be a hazard to your health) or your office building (which may be loaded with potentially harmful substances) for possible toxic chemicals.

CHEMICAL CFS

The Environmental Protection Association of the United States has found that the concentration of some toxic chemicals in ordinary homes and office buildings is some 200 to 500 per cent higher than that in the outside air. This is why the health problems this causes are sometimes referred to as the 'Sick Building Syndrome'. The problem is people tend to associate the word building with office blocks, skyscrapers, etc., without realising their humble abode is, at least for the purpose of such studies, a 'building'.

Common sources of pollutants are adhesives, carpeting, vinyl or rubber moulding, pressed wood, copying machines, cooking gas, cleaning agents and pesticides. There is little doubt in my mind that these can cause or aggravate a variety of conditions, including CFS.

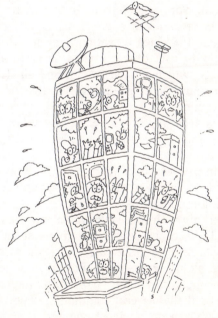

People who are very sensitive or who are already overloaded are usually affected by the chemicals such buildings contain and tend to complain of headaches, irritated eyes, drowsiness, skin rashes, difficulty in breathing and a host of other allergy-related conditions. Worse, these acute symptoms may be followed years later by more severe health consequences. Formaldehyde, benzene and trichloroethylene — three of the most common indoor pollutants — are known to be able to re-activate dormant latent viruses and are suspected of being able to cause a variety of cancers.

According to United States government reports, indoor contaminants cost the nation tens of billions of dollars per year in lost productivity and medical bills.

There are many companies that can survey and test for everything from moulds and dust mites to toxic chemicals and electromagnetic radiation. A list of these can be found at the back of this book on page 246.

It goes without saying that good nutrition, ample supplies of antioxidants and avoidance of the worst offenders are basic steps. But there are other steps you can take. Find out everything you can about keeping your personal environment safe. As well you can take simple precautions such as using a special vacuum cleaner with a very fine filter, a heating element to kill dust mites, and a water flow to trap dust particles. You can also purchase 'wardrobe camels', which reduce mould, and air de-humidifiers. Also there are many 'safe' products available on the market, ranging from recycled paper, non-allergenic cosmetics, soaps and laundry detergents, as well as shower heads that remove chlorine and thus enable you to enjoy long hot showers. In addition you can try 'plant power'.

After spending twenty odd years testing all sorts of things, NASA has finally found a workable weapon in the war against indoor air pollution: plants!

Scientists working with space capsules always had to deal with small, cramped spaces in which astronauts spend long hours without fresh air. Space vehicles are full, I am sure, of gadgets that pollute the air. By exposing plants to high concentrations of different chemicals, William Wolverton, an environmental engineer, discovered that several common varieties of plants are able to gobble up a wide range of contaminants from benzene in tobacco smoke to formaldehyde in household cleaners. Aloe vera removed 90 per cent of the formaldehyde in the air; marginata reduced benzene by almost 80 per cent; and peace lily cut trichlorethyne by half.

Since no one plant can tackle all pollutants, Wolverton suggested cultivating a mix of plants that excels at breaking down different classes of compounds (see table). One or two plants per 10 square metres is usually sufficient, although severe problems may require air venting or removing pollutant sources as well.

To maximise anti-pollution capabilities, Wolverton developed a 'filter planter' — basically a high-tech flowerpot. The container holds a hydroponic growth medium — carbon and porous clay pebbles — that he says traps pollutants more effectively than ordinary soil.

Pollutant	Sources	Health risk	Plant solution
Formaldehyde	Foam insulation, plywood, clothes, carpeting, furniture, paper goods, household cleaners, cosmetics (rare), dyes	Headaches, irritation of eyes and/or upper respiratory tract, asthma, throat cancer (with prolonged exposure)	Philodendron, spider plant, golden pothos, corn plant, chrysanthemum, mother-in-law's tongue
Benzene	Tobacco smoke, gasoline, synthetic fibres, plastics, inks, oils, detergents, rubber	Irritation of skin and eyes, headaches, loss of appetite, drowsiness, leukaemia and other blood diseases	English ivy, marginata, chrysanthemum, gerbera daisy, warneckei, peace lily
Trichloro-ethylene	Dry-cleaning, inks, paints, varnishes, lacquers, adhesives	Cancer of the liver	Gerbera, chrysanthemum, peace lily, marginata, warneckei

AN ANTI-POLLUTION GUIDE THAT WILL MAKE YOU SMARTER

The more natural the diet, the less stress imposed on the organism. Therefore, all functions will benefit from a clean diet. Remember, a healthy mind can only exist in a healthy body! The abolition of junk foods, sugar, coloured foods and drinks, and the elimination or avoidance of all nutritional excesses will also benefit all individuals.

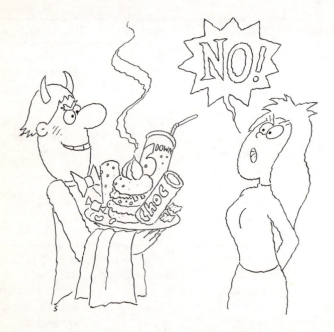

Many nutritional scientists have found that some vitamins help the brain to function close to its optimum. At the Institute for Orthomolecular Research I have often seen an improvement of mental ability occur as the result of treatment which involved megadoses of vitamins for other problems. Over the years the Institute has collected a veritable mass of scientific information to show the influence of these nutrients on the mind.

Getting smart or, at least, staying smart with nutrition is something which requires an understanding of the basic fact that, just as all cells of your body need nutrients to perform their various functions, so do the brain cells. Because the brain cells' functions involve thinking, anything that results in less than optimal nutrition for the cells will result in less than optimal thinking by the brain. Brain cells, again like all body cells, need to be constantly supplied with molecules derived from the food you eat. Most, if not all, brain chemicals (called neurotransmitters) are, in fact, made in the brain from precursors or amino acids supplied by the diet. What we call thinking, memory, concentration, etc., are in fact, functions of complex brain chemicals.

The metabolic rate of the whole body (brain included) is regulated by a gland called the thyroid. This gland is adversely affected by certain foods, and helped by iodine and kelp.

Vitamin C helps promote all cellular responses to hormones and should, therefore, always be included in any 'get smart' anti-pollution plan.

Glutamic acid has a special function in the brain; it picks up excessive ammonia from the brain cells. A form of glutamic acid, called glutamine, is particularly effective in this function, and it has been shown to improve thinking, clear the brains of alcoholics, reduce foggy minds during a hangover, and improve early morning alertness. So this one, too, could be very useful to students swatting for exams.

For vitamin C, eat plenty of peppers, capsicums, tomatoes and citrus fruits. Choline is available in wholegrains, beans (particularly soya beans, best eaten sprouted) or as lecithin capsules or granules and cold pressed oils like sunflower, safflower and sesame. Most of these foods also contain B6, magnesium and zinc. Eat plenty of nuts and seafood as well.

To be on the safe side, take a multi-vitamin supplement to support your good, varied, well-balanced diet.

Illnesses and Complications Associated with CFS

Allergies and CFS

WHY ME?
Why should people suffering from CFS be allergic? Worse still: why should someone who's NEVER been bothered by allergies, suddenly acquire an intolerance to common foods like wheat, milk or chocolate pudding? Why, after growing up with gas cooking and heating, should anyone become sensitive to the smallest gas leak? And of course, one may wonder why an allergy which has not caused much trouble since childhood should flare up all of a sudden. Yet all this happens quite often with CFS as it does with people who suffer other problems, notably candida infections.

Put simply, what happens is that when viral attacks begin, our immune system often panics. It starts to send out antibodies against everything it can think of. Substances that are usually only an irritation, such as dust or pollens, substances that contain potentially toxic components in minute and usually harmless quantities (salicylates in apples, solanine in tomatoes, etc.), all of a sudden have antibodies made against them, and become antigens, thus causing an allergic reaction of one kind or another. Perfumes, tobacco smoke, traffic pollution, insect sprays and even household detergents and ordinary paint can become a problem. Occasionally, the immune system may even make antibodies against parts of the body, causing all sorts of additional trouble (autoimmune disease).

Think of it this way: say someone threw a bomb in the middle of a crowded city. Chances are the police, bomb squad and who knows who else, would rush to the scene. It is probable that, in the confusion, the police would start to arrest anyone and everyone who even looked suspicious, whether he/she had anything to do with the bombing or not. This is how our immune system sometimes reacts.

Such intolerances that occur can be against almost anything, including of course chemicals. Hence the difficulty in separating some of these causes and effects when trying to establish whether CFS is of chemical or viral origin.

The immune system ties up these 'enemies' in groups and puts them on hold, as it were. Just like police cars responding to a headquarters radio call for assistance when a siege is underway, the body sends more and more soldiers (antibodies and white blood cells) to the places where those lumps are held. Meanwhile the system rounds up more and more suspects, making more and more lumps. The tissues where the lumps are located are soon swollen with them and begin to send alarm signals of their own. Histamine is released, neutrophils run around and the tissues become red, swollen and sore.

Other protective mechanisms come to help. Certain body surfaces start to make more mucus to trap and wash away all this stuff; the eyes water and swell for the same reason and one may start to cough or sneeze or have diarrhoea as the body tries to expel the mess. Once this has happened, the 'memory' of the immune system will code all the factors as enemies and when you are in contact with them again, you have an allergic attack, again and again. It is as if the body takes out its revenge on dust, pollens, moulds, gluten or whatever, for the harm viruses have inflicted upon it.

DEFINITION OF 'ALLERGY'

Although a dictionary (Webster's) defines allergy as 'an exaggerated or pathological reaction to substances, situations or physical states that are without comparable effect on the average individual', you would be surprised at the incredible disagreement which exists among scientists on the meaning of that term. To the majority of medical practitioners 'allergy' is only a reaction which involves the body's immune system and can be measured to provoke a particular response by certain antibodies, particularly immunoglobulin E (IgE). What most people call an allergy may be given other names by some medical scientists: idiosyncratic reaction, hypersensitivity, and intolerance are some of the words used.

This is why your GP may insist that your colitis is not really an allergy, in spite of the fact that whenever you eat a particular food your stomach feels like a band of gremlins have taken it over for a game of soccer. Many professionals are trying to abandon the term 'allergy' and prefer the less precise term 'intolerance'. By whatever name, it makes very little difference to the sufferer except perhaps when it comes to finding out exactly to what he or she is allergic. Even when you do find out, the problem remains of just how many and which foods, in any given groups, you should avoid, not to mention for how long.

THE CHANGING FACE OF ALLERGY

An allergy is simply an unusual reaction to something that would not normally bother the majority of individuals. At its most basic level it is caused by a reaction to certain unfriendly or threatening factors in the environment.

In order to have an allergy one has to become sensitised to the allergen. Everybody is exposed to dust every day and dust is an irritant, but only some people are allergic to it.

So there is a difference between an irritation, such as tears when someone blows smoke in your eyes, and an allergy, which involves a number of immunological and biochemical responses.

Because there is a well-established link between our immune system and all other body systems, including the brain (nervous system), allergies can cause almost any imaginable reaction. Just as a chain will break first at its weakest link, so an allergic person will show symptoms in his/her weakest element.

Contrary to popular belief, *Candida albicans,* the yeast fungus that causes thrush, is not only a potential trigger of allergies, but can be an allergen on its own. For more information see Allergies to Candida on p. 155.

Allergies are often associated with addictions to (cravings for) the allergen, but this is usually only in the case of foods. Inhalant/environmental allergies almost invariably make the sufferer feel 'uneasy' or unwell when exposed to the allergen.

Allergies that exist from childhood are often hereditary and avoidance of the allergen, such as a special elimination or anti-allergy diet, will not cure the allergy at all. It will simply remove the triggers for an allergic reaction. Unfortunately this can make a person even more sensitive, so that when they are accidentally exposed to the allergen, they will suffer even more than before. There are many ways to test for this and treatment can be via special vaccines (sublingual), desensitisation (injections) or neutralisation (intradermal serial dilution titration). Naturally, avoidance is also practised as far as possible.

The most important vitamins, minerals and other supplements for allergies vary greatly, depending on the type of allergy and what one is allergic to. Zinc, for example, while helpful, will not be as efficient as magnesium if the allergy is to a chemical such as perfume, insecticides, household cleaners, etc.

People who develop allergies all of a sudden, often do so because of exposure to a latent virus — one that does not necessarily cause any serious symptoms or perhaps is mistaken for a bad cold or a flu. The Epstein Barr is one such virus. Because it takes up permanent residence in a part of our immune system (the B-cells), it can remain dormant for years on end. If activated, it causes a 'panic' situation and the body will begin to make antibodies to everything and anything that looks vaguely suspicious. One then enters the same dusty room one has inhabited for years, gets out the vacuum cleaner and pronto! An allergy is born. Cure the underlying viral condition and the allergy promptly disappears.

Exposure to chemicals, even low-grade exposure over a long period of time, can cause allergies. Someone can live in a house that has mould under the floorboards for years without being affected. Then he/she goes to work in a highly polluted office, or has the house repainted or has the pest controllers in for spiders. The chemical residuals linger on and, after a time, the individual begins to have strange symptoms such as a sudden need for a lot more sleep, headaches, poor concentration and mood swings.

Removing the chemicals, by a thorough detoxification of the house, will not help because as long as the mould remains under the floorboards, the hapless individual, who is by now severely allergic to it, will not improve.

On the other hand, removing the mould, while obviously helping for a while, will not cure the problem because the continuing exposure to chemical residuals will ensure the patient becomes allergic to the next thing he/she is exposed to.

In addition, we now know that food particles (allergenic proteins) can be absorbed via the small intestine in undigested form. Some pass through the blood to the brain and thus enter the nervous system. These 'allergenic foods' can disrupt immune functions and the nervous system. If one realises that these two systems are interwoven and interact all the time, it is easy to see that allergies can be one of the causes of CFS-like illness, as well as being a common symptom of CFS sufferers.

Allergies are associated with an underactive immune system but sometimes hyperactivity of the immune system is the underlying biochemical problem. This is why we now refer simply to immune dysregulation, rather than to one or the other. Fortunately, there are a number of blood tests, admittedly rather sophisticated, that can tell us not only if the immune system is under-, or overactive, but also WHICH part of the immune system is at fault.

FOOD FAMILIES

To the lay person, a tomato is quite different to a potato and few non-professionals would see a connection between tomato sauce, fruit juices and cakes, although they all contain yeast moulds/fungi. You see, although people talk about 'food' allergies or intolerances, most patients are not sensitive to the foods as such but rather to some natural or added chemical or other which in most cases is common to a food family.

The potato, for example, is one member of the nightshade family, as are tomatoes, capsicums, eggplants and tobacco. All these contain solanine, a natural chemical which is potentially toxic and to which many people are very sensitive. In fact, some nutritional scientists claim that an intolerance, or allergy, to nightshades is one of the commonest causes of arthritis. In addition all these foods also contain nicotine, so that it is possible, although not common, for some to be allergic to tobacco and therefore to be affected by eating some of these foods.

In other cases, people may not be allergic to any component of the foods but rather to something extraneous to it, like the moulds which grow on tea leaves, dried fruit, cream cheese, melons and indeed on most leftovers which are allowed to stay in the fridge overnight. From here on things become even more complicated. Some people are allergic to wheat. This could mean that they are hypersensitive to gluten. Some gluten-sensitive patients may also need to avoid non-grain foods which contain gluten, such as buckwheat, cassava, arrowroot and tapioca. They can eat rice, both brown and white, as well as millet and corn, however, because these grains are gluten-free. On the other hand, some people appear to be sensitive to some factor in grains other than gluten. In most such cases, these patients cannot eat rice, millet, wheat, rye, oats, barley, malt and corn although buckwheat, cassava, arrowroot and tapioca are allowed.

Then there is the special problem of corn. Apart from its potential allergenicity as part of the grains group, this food appears to exert its own special kind of intolerance. Most commercial adhesives and also talcum powder can thus provoke a reaction in a corn-sensitive patient.

Just as Ben Feingold mistakenly postulated that all hyperactive children were only sensitive to chemical additives and salicylates, without giving any consideration to the twin possibilities of lowered immunocompetence caused by vitamin and mineral deficiencies and the likelihood of allergies to other common foods, so, many investigators have fallen for the trap of cutting off potential reactions by postulating different degrees of allergenicity for individual members of each food family.

So you will hear and read learned pronouncements about wheat being more allergenic than rice, when, in fact, all one can say is that, statistically, there are less people with an intolerance to rice than to wheat, which is due to the fact that there are more people sensitive to gluten than to other grain factors. Having said that, I must admit that not all members of a particular food family need necessarily cause reaction in all allergic patients. The problem is to know who is sensitive to what, and how much. Obviously one would not be able to correlate the enormous variations possible within even a relatively small group of patients, so there are only two practical answers.

First, one must have a detailed medical history which, in the hands of an experienced therapist, will often elicit some important information. We do know that there are some valid generalisations. Statistically, more people are allergic to eggs than to chicken, to soya than to lentils, so one starts with at least some idea of what is more likely to cause harm. The family history will also provide some clues as will the actual presenting symptoms because, once again, there are some statistical correlations between certain food intolerances and body systems that tend to be affected by them. So milk and dairy products often have the respiratory tract as a target, while grains feature more prevalently in digestive problems.

Many trials, some double blind, have shown that some patients react to one member of a food family show no reaction at all when challenged by another member of the same family. So it is possible that one may feel unwell after eating tomatoes, but can munch away at potatoes every day without feeling any different. In fact all sorts of patients react to various combinations of foods in ways that can only be ascribed to biochemical individuality.

Then there is the problem of not knowing whether the lack of reaction is simply due to the fact that the patient eats one or the other food less often, or more often, than other members of the same food family. Finally, the absence of any visible or subjective reaction does not altogether exclude the possibility that the food may, in fact, be harmful.

In addition, the individual's resistance varies from day to day, and even from hour to hour. Because the first dictum of health professionals is 'Thou shalt do no harm', the only way is to play safe, and ask the patient's body, by monitoring its subtle signals, if the ingestion of a particular food is stressful .

HYPOGLYCAEMIA, FOOD CRAVINGS AND ALLERGIES/INTOLERANCES

After many years, during which most nutritionists treated hypoglycaemia (fluctuating blood sugar levels) and the food cravings associated with it, as a disease, we have now realised that it is but a symptom of deeper, underlying metabolic problems. One of the most common causes of hypoglycaemia is an unsuspected food intolerance/allergy.

The differential diagnosis of this problem is quite simple. Generally a person who has a food allergy will feel better when fasting, while a true hypoglycaemic is more likely to feel unwell. One simple test is to perform a glucose tolerance test (GTT) with a suspected food, instead of the customary glucose. If blood sugars increase, or drop out of proportion to the type of food eaten, then the likelihood is that that patient is reacting to the food, because the body interprets the ingestion as a form of stress. This causes the release of stress hormones and these tend to produce elevations in blood sugar levels, often followed by a rapid drop, until the cravings drive one to ingest more of the offending food. Thus, many food cravings and even binges are created.

ALLERGY TESTING

There are many ways of testing allergies. Skin scratch tests are one of the most common ways but, in order to be effective they have to be followed (after several hours at least) by an end pointing procedure. This allows the therapist to prepare a suitable vaccine for the allergies in the form of sublingual drops. Other tests, called RAST, can ferret out allergies to some chemicals, as well as some foods. Then there are a number of testing procedures with 'challenges' as well as a method called serial dilution titration neutralisation, which is rather complex but can be very effective in difficult cases. Another, called the 'patch' test, allows us to uncover skin sensitivities to a number of chemical agents.

All this makes the treatment much more effective and it eliminates one of the dangers of boosting immunity in someone who is allergic before knowing what the underlying problem is.

This is very important, so *please note carefully* that a number of severe conditions, known as autoimmune diseases, are caused by an overactive, gone-crazy immune response. Although in many cases there is a genetic (hereditary) predisposition for these ailments, it is quite possible to precipitate such a condition, or aggravate an existing one, by overstimulating immunity with inappropriate treatments. Fortunately this will be reflected quickly and quite clearly in the tests one uses to monitor such procedures—so the therapist can alter the treatment immediately.

There are several tests for allergies — some are more valid than others. These tests include the pulse test, which tests for pulse rate elevation on exposure to allergens (pulse rate may vary for other reasons such as exposure to indoor environmental pollutants); tests to monitor the changes in the body's ascorbic acid levels, which decrease when the body is under stress; tests of the saliva pH content, which indicates whether the metabolic acidosis that often follows an acute allergic reaction has occurred; and muscle kinesiology tests, which measure the changes in muscle strength after the ingestion of allergenic foods. These tests are generally valid if carried out carefully, but should not be used for diagnosis on their own. Avoidance–challenge tests indicate allergies by the reaction to allergens either by fasting and challenging or by avoiding and challenging and are simple and useful if carefully conducted; the cytotoxic test, which tests for foods that may be poisonous or toxic to the cells in your body is expensive and controversial; and the RAST (Radio Allergo Sorbent Test), which measures the specific antibody's (IgE) response to suspect food fragments, is sometimes useful as a diagnostic tool and is an excellent preventative test.

DUST MITES AND FUNGI

It is a sad but true fact that what may start off in the early life of a child as recurrent colds, skin rashes, oral thrush, ear infections, bronchial congestions, milk allergy or colic can sometimes become a respiratory illness such as asthma in later life. Such a state of affairs may, in the long term, weaken or disrupt the immune system, leaving the way open for viral infections, chemical sensitivities and other problems that may lead to CFS later in life.

There is mounting evidence that exposure to dust mites, moulds and a variety of other toxins and allergens during early childhood can predispose children to asthma and other allergic diseases in later life.

We know that asthma is an allergic disease and that many different factors can trigger an asthma attack. One can be sparked by such diverse events as stress, viral illness, sudden changes of climate and/or temperature, not to mention exercise, etc.

But the basic, underlying *cause* of many respiratory ailments, such as asthma, sinusitis, hay fever and chronic bronchial congestion is often an allergy. The individual is, in other words, unusually sensitive to something that normally does not affect other people at the same dose or exposure.

The most common respiratory disease allergens (factors that cause allergies) are dust mites, moulds, grasses and other pollens, some chemicals (like MSG and formaldehyde), food additives (especially sulphites and colourings), as well as many of the multitude of pollutants we spew into our atmosphere.

Consider the following statistics: Australia is experiencing an epidemic of asthma, which is now the fourth main cause of medical death in this country; 10 per cent of Australian adults and 20 per cent of Australian children suffer asthma; 75 per cent of deaths due to asthma occur in the over-fifty group; Australia has the dubious honour of having the world's second highest rate of asthma deaths (New Zealand is the first); between 1984 and 1988 the incidence of asthma case admission to Sydney's Prince of Wales Hospital for Children increased by 53 per cent; in 1990 more people died of asthma in Australia than of AIDS; yet experts say 95 per cent of asthmatics should lead a normal, wheeze-free life.

So what can you do to treat, alleviate and prevent asthma?

Dust mites

Dust mites cannot be seen with the naked eye. Yet chances are you feed and shelter between 250 000 and 1 million of them in your bed while you sleep, predisposing you to asthma and other allergic respiratory illnesses. In some cases they cause insomnia. And all it takes is 1 billionth of a gram of one.

How do you get rid of or control dust and dust mites? It goes without saying that keeping one's house clean and the bedroom super-clean will help. But often it is not as easy as that. To start with, many allergic people will be sensitised by the invisible particles of dust which escape at great velocity from vacuum cleaners. And the dust mites IN the vacuum cleaner can easily find their way back to you when you try to clean the instrument, although there are some vacuum cleaners on the market that will kill the mites by cooking them as it were. And many vacuum cleaners are not strong enough to suck all the allergens from deep within mattresses. And far too many people have carpets in the house and bedroom. (Asthmatics and allergy sufferers in general should avoid carpets and NEVER sleep in carpeted bedrooms.)

Fungi

Fungi (the word is synonymous with 'moulds') are everywhere and because in Australia we generally live in a warm, humid climate, we are wading through a sea of them. Although fungi have enjoyed a symbiotic relationship with humans for millennia, in recent years there has been an explosion of fungal infections and intolerances (allergies). There is little doubt now that moulds can cause, trigger or contribute to a wide range of illnesses.

Although the best known mould is *Candida albicans*, a yeast fungus that usually causes thrush (either systemic or vaginal), there are many other disease-causing moulds, with some being more toxic than others. Irrespective of the causes, the fact is that a depressed immune system favours both the growth/proliferation and toxicity of fungi. The fungi themselves are often immunosuppressive, thus compounding the effects.

Asthma, indeed many respiratory and allergic diseases, can be caused, triggered or aggravated by moulds (dust mites often contain moulds) and xenobiotics (chemicals). In addition, medical researchers found that people living in damp homes are more likely to become sick than those living in dry, mould-free houses. Allergies, inexplicable bouts of fatigue, lethargy, sleep problems, sore throats, runny noses, wheezing, fevers, headaches, dizziness, mood swings, insomnia and mental confusion have all been associated with the presence of moulds.

Just as in the case of dust mites, one can't always see moulds. They may be growing unabated for months giving off toxic spores before anyone becomes aware of their existence.

For several years now, we have been using a number of methods for assessing the presence of moulds and dust mites in our patients' bedrooms. Since using these methods, I have noted a remarkable coincidence between the number and types of mould found and some of our patients' health, as well as their ability to recover from a variety of illnesses.

Recently scientists have also developed facilities to eradicate or control both dust mites and moulds. This has been incredibly successful. Indeed, after we have arranged for the eradication of mould and dust mites from their bedroom, many of our patients find that all manner of seemingly unrelated symptoms disappear or diminish dramatically and they get a good night's sleep and wake up refreshed for the first time in years.

Apart from the potential toxicity of the moulds themselves, recent studies have found that some fungi give off dust fumes that can cause toxic reactions.

It all comes back to the simple and obvious principle of 'total load'. When you go to bed at night, you get (hopefully) some rest. If you are sensitive to moulds and dust mites, your immune system does not get any respite. By the time you wake up, half your energy has been spent fighting the ubiquitous blights.

Strong sunlight tends to kill mites and fungi. So does heat. In fact, if you could heat the interior of your house to about 50°C you would kill cockroaches, mites, flies, ticks, moths and even termites. Believe it or not, in California (where else?) there is already a pest control firm appropriately called 'Isothermic', which completely treats homes, with no chemical in sight, using just that, heat. In addition, there are a number of preparations on the market that kill and control dust mites as well as moulds. They have to be applied carefully and are usually sold with a full set of instructions. An average bedroom can take a couple of hours of hard work.

Candida and CFS

Many, if not most, CFS sufferers have a problem with candida. They either carry a candida infection or are allergic to *Candida albicans* or other forms of yeast fungi (moulds). In fact, I believe that candida can, and often does, cause chronic fatigue. If you are always tired and have a candida problem, then the candida organism may be the cause. Yet if your CFS is caused by something other than candida then it is very likely to trigger a candida explosion. Indeed the candida organism's effect on you may well prevent any treatment for CFS being successful, and so the candida problem must be taken care of as part of the treatment for CFS.

CANDIDA — WHAT IT IS AND WHAT IT IS NOT
Many people are confused by candida. It is not the name of a disease, it is part of the name of an organism that is responsible for many health problems. The full name of the organism is *Candida albicans,* of which there are many varieties, strains and

types. Candida is a yeast fungus and therefore a candida infection is sometimes known as a yeast infection. When people think of yeast infections they immediately think of thrush or monilia — which mean the same thing and which are generally associated with vaginal thrush. This condition was first described by Hippocrates some 2000 years ago.

Many women are familiar with the symptoms of vaginal thrush (or monilia or vaginal candidiasis): the itchiness, even soreness, swelling, and the white, often odorous discharge (from which *Candida albicans* gets the second part of its name: *alba* means white).

However, many different parts of the body can be affected by candidiasis in localised infections: the nails, mouth, skin, ears, genitals, rectum, etc. Or it can be systemic, meaning that candida, or one of the several dozen toxins it can spawn, can invade one or more body systems, such as the circulatory system, the respiratory system or the digestive system. Systemic candidiasis can affect any part, organ or system of the body without the symptoms of vaginal thrush even being present.

And this is where the problem lies. Too many doctors will tell someone suffering from vaginal thrush that it is only 'a bit of a nuisance', and that it can be cleared up with some cream. But such treatments only attack the symptoms of the candida infection locally. What they don't take account of is that a candida infection might appear in localised symptoms, but the real problem is focussed not in the vagina, the mouth, or wherever, it is focussed in the intestine, where the organism has grown unchecked by competing bacteria or the body's own defences in the immune system. Therefore for candida to be treated properly, the local symptoms must of course be attacked, but so should the problem as a whole. If you don't cure the problem in the gut the likelihood of local recurrences is enormous. So, next time your doctor decides to treat your candida problem topically (that is, in the location of the obvious symptoms), remind him that it is impossible to have a localised infection without having a candida problem in the gut at the same time. BOTH AREAS SHOULD BE TREATED, or you will never get rid of it. In fact it says exactly this in an article that appeared in the *Journal of the American Medical Association* (Vol. 238, No. 17):

> ... vaginal candidiasis does not occur naturally without the concurrent presence of *Candida albicans* within the large bowel ... a cure is not likely as long as the vagina remains the only target of treatment. There is no evidence that *Candida albicans*, once it becomes part of the fecal flora, ever leaves the host [that's *you*] spontaneously during his or her lifetime ... A cure for candidiasis would not be possible without the prior eradication of *Candida albicans* from the gut ...

What this means is that if you, your partner or children have ever had any form of thrush even once in your lifetime, your digestive system has been affected. Unless you have been prescribed oral antifungals at the time, the condition will never have gone completely away, thus making you prone to recurrence if your immune defences become low.

WHY YOU MIGHT HAVE CANDIDA

Many doctors and therapists use questionnaires as part of their diagnostic procedure for candidiasis. While many of the questions asked are useful pointers, it should always be remembered that the specific symptoms may also be the result of other illnesses, hereditary allergies or a depressed immune system. Here are the most commonly asked questions in diagnostic questionnaires, for which I have also added an analysis in brackets. Candidiasis may be a cause of, or a serious component of, your health problems if:

1. You have ever had vaginal thrush, particularly if it was only treated topically (locally). (This is invariably valid in establishing at least the possibility of candida playing a part in your health problems.)
2. You have taken antibiotics, particularly of the broad-spectrum variety, many times during childhood and again later on. (This, too, is valid, although not as categorical as point 1. Broad spectrum antibiotics can allow candida infestations to develop because they can affect the ability of your body's natural defence mechanisms to attack the candida organism.)

3   You have suffered from recurrent ear infections, tinea, athlete's foot, nail infections (paronichia), skin rashes, oral thrush, colic, jock itch, or allergies during infancy, childhood, or since. (This can be a good indication, but it should be remembered that these symptoms can also point to other illnesses or allergies.)
4   Your problems started after taking an oral contraceptive. (This is often a valid point, unless the problem is hormonal.)
5   You are, or have been, pregnant and symptoms of vaginal thrush have appeared. (This is usually a valid point.)
6   You suffer from any type of pre-menstrual syndrome (there are at least five). (This is valid, too, but other causes may be such problems as APICH, thyroid problems, hormonal imbalances, etc.)
7   You have suffered from pelvic inflammatory disease (PID) or from endometriosis. (PID and endometriosis may be caused by a variety of factors and, if no cause has been found for their occurrence, the symptoms may actually be due to undiagnosed candidiasis.)
8   You have had recurring nasal polyps. (Common enough in males, this factor is more often due to a respiratory allergy to moulds than to a candida infection, although it remains a possibility.)
9   You have been treated with immuno-suppressive drugs such as steroids, cortisone or predinisone for skin problems, asthma, arthritis, etc. (A very valid point provided one makes sure that any possible side effects of the drugs have been excluded as the problem.)
10 Your symptoms seem to be aggravated when you eat yeast or food containing moulds. (A valid point, but it is essential to differentiate between allergy and infection.)
11 Your symptoms tend to come on or get worse during wet weather, on humid days, or when exposed to dampness. (More valid than point 10, but again, it can be a sign of an allergy/intolerance to moulds. This is especially so if the symptoms involve the ears, nose, throat or chest and manifests as sinusitis, asthma or hay fever.)
12 You feel tired on damp days or after working in the garden on wet days. (As above.)

13 You are uncomfortable around chemical pollutants such as cigarette smoke, petrol fumes, gas used in stoves and heaters, insecticides, perfumes, etc. (Not a valid point as such sensitivity is very common in much more serious conditions such as Chronic Fatigue Syndrome, Universal Reactivity Syndrome, chemical overloading/allergy, Post-viral Syndrome, Chronic Epstein Barr, and, of course, environmental illnesses. Candida is a very common symptom of all these conditions. Having said that, please remember that it is possible for *Candida albicans* to facilitate, trigger or provoke these conditions as well.)

14 You experience recurrent cravings for sweets, alcohol and carbohydrates. (Not particularly valid as cravings tend to be associated with many other conditions such as allergies — one tends to crave what one is allergic to — or hypoglycaemia.)

15 You suffer from depression. (Not a valid point as depression may be emotional, a reaction to being ill all the time, or be caused by a very wide range of conditions ranging from vitamin B12 deficiency, a lack of sunshine, chemical overloading, and everything in between.)

16 You are continually tired for no reason. (Almost invariably invalid by itself as chronic tiredness can be caused by so many other factors.)

17 You have problems concentrating, remembering things and have a general feeling of being 'spaced out'. (Often associated with chronic systemic or intestinal thrush, it is common, however, in many other conditions.)

18 You have problems controlling your weight. (While it is true that candida sufferers have weight problems, it is equally true that one can be overweight, as well as tired, as a result of a low thyroid condition, poor liver clearance of oestrogen, and at least a dozen other reasons.)

19 You experience recurring sore throats, nasal congestion, hay fever, sinusitis or ear infections. (These symptoms are associated with candida but may also point to Post-viral Syndrome, CFS and allergies.)

20 If you crave or prefer yeast-derived foods or foods that contain yeast such as cheeses, beer, wines, commercial fruit

juices, vinegar, etc. (These cravings are common in cases of intestinal thrush that feature a lot of associated energy and 'mental' problems.)

21 You find sweets give you a 'lift' but then you feel worse later on. (Always associated with hypoglycaemia and allergies, this reaction does not necessarily involve candida problems.)

In addition, multiple pregnancies, chronic or repeated infections, recurrent cystitis, the loss of libido (sexual desire) and skin problems are signs of possible candida infestation or sensitisation.

As you can see from the list above, all these factors may point to possible candidiasis, but many point just as much to other illnesses. None alone can point to a candidiasis problem. While questionnaires can establish a connection between your health problems and *Candida albicans,* what they may not necessarily be able to do is differentiate between candida as a *cause* or candida as a *symptom* of your illness. So it is essential that your doctor or therapist takes a thorough medical history, too.

It should also be remembered that *Candida albicans* is an opportunistic organism, and can create problems even when something entirely different has *caused* your illness by upsetting your body in general and your immunity in particular. A lot of time can be wasted in treating candida which is only a symptom and not the underlying cause of your ill health. Of course you may initially feel better if your treatment is directed at candida because it may remove the symptoms. But, particularly if the treatment is by diet alone, this could occur if the problem was actually caused by allergies, hypoglycaemia or a nutritional imbalance.

SYMPTOMS OF CANDIDA INFECTION
Apart from the vaginal/genital symptoms associated with thrush, candida can cause a wide variety of symptoms. Broadly speaking they fall predominantly into the following groups:

Digestive symptoms
Loose bowels • diarrhoea/constipation • excessive flatus • irritable bowel • malabsorption • abdominal bloating • heartburn • nausea.

Mucocutaneous (affecting the mucous membranes throughout the body) symptoms
Thrush • skin rashes • ear/nose/mouth/vaginal/rectal infections • inflammation or irritation • discharges • itching • nail infections and itchiness.
Emotional/mental symptoms
PMS (pre-menstrual syndromes) • anxiety • depression • agoraphobia • nervousness • short temper • poor concentration.
Allergic symptoms
Sinusitis • hay fever • post-nasal drip • throat mucus • headaches • skin rashes • sneezing • chest/bronchial congestion • asthma.

ALLERGIES TO CANDIDA

There is considerable controversy about whether *Candida albicans* infections can affect immunity. In many cases it is not clear if someone has a candida problem or not. An individual can have a candida infection without being allergic to the candida organism; or he/she can be very allergic without having an infection. Sometimes the individual has an infection *and* is allergic. An allergy to candida can result in a variety of symptoms which may involve organs and glands anywhere in the body, even those remote from the areas that have been infected by the organism. It can be associated with foods, chemicals or environmental allergies/intolerances or sensitivities, as well as dysfunctions of many glands and therefore hormone and enzyme systems. It can also cause heart problems. Such a condition is known as Chronic Candidiasis Sensitivity Syndrome.

Symptoms of candida allergy/intolerance
The symptoms of a candida allergy are similar to those of allergies/intolerances to moulds/fungi — with one exception: the so-called 'die-off' reaction can last longer and be severe enough to impede treatment if an infection is present at the same time.

'Die-off' occurs when, during antifungal treatment, the dying candida organisms are reabsorbed and, because they change and release toxins, this can cause a worsening of the symptoms. If the patient is allergic to moulds the reaction will be more severe and last longer. In addition, treatment to desensitise any allergy to moulds/fungi or candida may actually cause a reaction instead of alleviating the symptoms. It is therefore important to know whether someone is allergic or not because it affects the treatment

— whether diet and herbal remedies will be used alone, whether desensitisation to moulds is begun after the treatment is completed, whether the treatment should be changed, etc.

EXAMINATION, TESTS AND DIAGNOSIS

We have already seen that a questionnaire is a useful although not conclusive tool in determining whether someone is suffering from candida. It is also essential that a complete medical history be collected. A thorough physical examination is also very helpful. *All* potential locations should be carefully examined. It is not just a matter, as some doctors tell their patients, of 'taking a quick look' at the vagina of someone who has vaginal thrush. Some patients may suffer from candida which has not localised in the vagina and therefore will show no symptoms there. Remember, a candida/yeast infection does not just equal vaginal thrush or monilia alone.

No single test is sufficient for a full identification of the whole candida species or for telling whether a candida intolerance exists. There are several methods, however, that have been used for diagnosis. The blood cells analysis (variously known as 'live cell analysis', 'live blood analysis', 'darkfield analysis' among others) is a relatively new method of viewing a blood sample obtained by the finger-prick method. It is then possible to report on a number of measurements and observations of blood cells and parameters. In my experience and that of many of my colleagues this test has little value. The presence of *Candida albicans* does not necessarily mean that it will make you ill, because the organism may not be pathogenic, may not adhere to tissue surfaces (unless it does it will cause no harm) and your body may be taking care of it anyway.

Other tests include the VEGA test, which would appear to be very subjective and useful only in the hands of a very experienced practitioner; the IgE, RAST (radio-allergo absorbent test), skin scratch and endpointing tests, which will indicate whether someone is allergic to candida and to a range of other moulds and fungi, as well as indicating whether a patient's immune system is capable of mounting a defence against the organism; and the CMI (cell mediated immunity) test, which is also known as a multitest, and includes candida as one of a number of challenges applied under the skin (it is an excellent test not only for candida but also for ascertaining whether a patient's immunity is the problem; it identifies those patients with very poor immunity and they are the ones most likely to suffer from chronic candida infections and allergies, as well as CFS and other health problems).

If candida is present, as it is in most people, then it must be found out if it is harming the body. If it is, then there will be an antibody response. This can be measured accurately with a candida antibodies test. However, if the body cannot make antibodies, or if the antibodies are all busy attaching themselves to the candida organisms, then you can't measure anything. So, first the antibodies should be checked. Irrespective of the results (that is, even iff perfectly normal) one then administers antifungal medications that one knows for sure will kill the organisms. Then one counts the antibodies to candida again. If their number has increased or decreased, then the diagnosis of candida infection is a reasonable one. In addition, one can run allergy tests for candida and associated moulds to ascertain if there is an allergy to candida.

Another useful test, this time for vaginal thrush, is a culture test (Sabourad's medium) which is accurate if performed under the correct conditions. It should be remembered, however, that this test will only reveal whether or not *Candida albicans* is present in the vagina, which may actually be totally free of candida while the colon or other areas of the body are heavily infested.

A further useful method of diagnosis is a trial elimination diet. Eliminating moulds, fungi and ferments, as well as nutrients that contribute to the growth of candida, such as refined carbohydrates, should improve a patient's condition. If it does not, then either the candida problem is more than superficial and will need more vigorous treatment, or there are other reasons for whatever symptoms one has. If the diet is successful in eliminating the problem, or at least in making one feel better, then a good result has been achieved. Unfortunately one would still not know whether candida was the problem or whether the patient was simply allergic to one of the foods avoided in the elimination diet.

The next simplest diagnostic procedure is to start a trial of anti-fungals, preferably specific anti-candida fungicides, to see if the patient improves. Again, if the patient improves all is well and, in such cases, a clear indication that candida was indeed a problem. The pitfalls with such a procedure, though, are many.

TREATMENTS

The first step in helping anyone with a suspected candida problem is to place them on a trial elimination diet. What kind of elimination diet, in other words what the diet eliminates, has to be decided after a full medical history has been taken and an examination of all the factors involved has been carried out. The reason for doing this is simple. Let us say someone has a raging *Candida albicans* overgrowth, which we know can upset the body's immunity and cause an individual to become allergic. Let us assume that in this case the patient has become allergic to salycilates, or rice, or whatever. They are then prescribed lots of fresh vegetable juices, a vitamin C supplement with bioflavonoids to help the absorption of the vitamin, plus brown rice. The patient will feel worse almost immediately. How would the therapist know if this was caused by a die-off reaction or an allergy or a lack of proteins or a thyroid problem, or whether the original symptoms had been caused by something else? Thus you can see that a full examination of all available information is essential.

But before we get on to what actually constitutes an elimination diet, I should mention Nystatin powder. In my clinical experience with thousands of candida cases I have found that starting the course of treatment with pure Nystatin powder is safer, faster and less likely to cause confusion than anything else. The reasons are simple. Nystatin is not absorbed into the body. It kills candida organisms on contact only, rather like pouring Draino down the sink. It will scour the inner tubes of the plumbing without affecting the tubes themselves. The Draino then leaves your plumbing system without entering your water supply. In much the same way Nystatin will not enter the blood and will be excreted quite safely.

When using Nystatin in your treatment remember that the powder should be pure and contain no preservatives, colourings or excipients (inert substances). Nystatin or Mycostatin capsules and tablets contain lactose and/or corn starch (which can be classed as excipients), as well as additives, so any reactions you may have had to Nystatin in the past might have been due to these factors.

Although the usual maintenance dose ranges from a quarter to half a teaspoon three to four times daily, you may need as much as one level teaspoon three to six times daily. If you have a concurrent allergy to moulds you should start with a low dose and work up to the full dose gradually.

Dissolve the powder in half to a full glass of distilled water or fresh vegetable juice. For maximum benefit you should take it one hour before meals but if this is too difficult take it with your meals. Swish the first mouthful around your mouth, retain for a minute, then swallow. Then drink the remainder.

Your therapist will tailor your dosage to you. Improvement of your symptoms and the results of tests will determine the dosage and timing that are right for you. In general, maintain the dose that alleviates gastric symptoms like bloating, diarrhoea, wind, heartburn, etc. Although Nystatin is quite safe, some people may experience an initial reaction, often due to an overload of the dying candida organism (die-off) or because they are allergic to candida. This should subside in a few days. If you become concerned about any reaction, please call your therapist.

Nystatin can also be made into a solution to use for gargling if your throat has been affected by candida, for swabbing your ears (many people suffering from candida experience recurrent ear infections or itchy ears). In that case it is advisable to swab your ears several times each day. The solution can also be used for hygenic precautions which I will outline later. Careful inhaling of pure Nystatin powder will help people with a variety of respiratory tract problems. To make up the Nystatin solution combine the following ingredients:

Half a litre (one pint) of lukewarm water
Full teaspoon of pure Nystatin powder
Two teaspoons of Cytobifidus (or a similar probiotic preparation)
Contents of one capsule of Caprinex (caprilic acid)
Five drops of essential fatty acid micelle (alternatively take one capsule of essential fatty acids)

This is the basic method for making the solution, although it may have to be tailored to individual requirements.

Nutritional requirements of *Candida albicans*

Candida's capacity to do harm is somehow linked with its ability to cling or adhere to the interior skin surface of tissues. Two distinct forms exist: the yeast form and the myceal form. This latter is apparent during invasive colonisation, but both are capable of causing symptoms and becoming pathogenic (doing harm). As well, both can change into any of some 15 different forms within a few months.

Research has shown that the growth of candida is promoted by a variety of sugars and polysaccharides, particularly glucose, corn sugar and biotin (a Vitamin B complex). As well, the sugars promote the organism's ability to adhere and thus become harmful. The most active sugar in this is galactose (a milk sugar), followed by glucose, fructose (in fruits etc.), sucrose and maltose (in starches). This may well be one reason why it is often wise to avoid milk products if you are infected by candida.

The ability of the organism to adhere is a measure of its toxicity, and some fatty acids block adherence, while others do not. Some combinations of nutrients can slow the growth of candida but increase its adherence. Your therapist will be able to tell you which foods to avoid.

Copper increases the virulence of the myceal form and is yet another reason for avoiding tap water, which often has a high copper content.

The vitamin and amino acid (the building blocks of proteins) requirements of *Candida albicans* have been extensively studied. *Candida albicans* and some of its varients need biotin, and some amino acids reduce the need for biotin. In fact, biotin is a double-edged sword: it encourages the increase of *Candida albicans* (its presence can help candida synthesize all the necessary amino acids for its survival and growth) while at the same time reducing its ability to change into the myceal form.

Antibiotics can create problems, as has already been mentioned. In people whose immune system has been weakened (such as organ transplant recipients, individuals on corticosteroids, or those undergoing intensive antibiotic therapy) the organism can spread systematically and even prove fatal. Antifungal drugs are generally very successful in killing the organisms, but it has also been discovered that too little anti-fungal medication given for too short a period of time can make the problem worse. Contrary to common belief some sulphur drugs (sulphonamides) can impare the body's ability to control and kill *Candida albicans*.

As I have already mentioned, *Candida albicans* comes in a yeast form. It is possible to be allergic to candida as well as infected by it, but as I explained earlier, you tend to crave the things you are allergic to. The following is a list of yeast products (sometimes known as leavened products), products containing moulds (fungi) and products containing ferments (the process of souring or fermentation):

Raised doughs   breads, rolls, buns, biscuits, cakes, pastries, all commercial baked goods
Vinegars   (apple, wine, pear, grape, etc.): includes all foods containing vinegar such as salad dressings, mayonnaise, pickles, sauerkrauts, olives, mince pies, and most condiments and sauces such as barbecue, tomato, chilli or pepper sauce
Fermented beverages   beer, wine, champagne, rum, brandy, tequila, root beer, ginger ale, as well as substances which contain alcohol, e.g. extracts, tinctures, cough mixtures and other medications
Cheeses   especially cottage cheese and including fermented dairy products such as yoghurt, buttermilk and sour cream
Malted products   malted milkshakes, some breakfast cereals, lollies, etc., which have been malted
Ferments and moulds   including soy sauce, truffles and mushrooms
Antibiotics   penicillin and most synthetic derivatives such as ampicillin, methecillin, amoxcillin and many other '-illins'

Other things to avoid include:
- Mycine drugs and related compounds such as erythromyacin, streptomycin, chloremphicol, tetracyclines, etc.
- All vitamins and health foods containing yeast, brewer's yeast and its derivatives
- All 'enriched' flours and special milk drinks that may have yeast added
- All cereals which have yeast added
- All commercial fruit drinks, tinned and frozen
- All cured meats such as salami, bacon, sausages, hot dogs, etc.

- Horseradish
- Almost all dried fruits
- Teas
- Miso
- Tofu
- Commercial nuts
- All melons
- Almost any leftover food placed in a refrigerator for as little as a few hours — so try to cook and prepare only what you are going to eat at each meal.

The Elimination Diet
This diet avoids most of the common allergens found in everyday foods, such as yeast, gluten grains, fungi, dairy products, preservatives, etc. You may only eat or drink things that are listed below — nothing else! Not only is this diet ideal for candidiasis, it also prepares you for any testing for possible allergies.

You will almost certainly lose weight but, a word of warning: because you may have become used to sugars, milk, yeast and other substances to the extent that you are actually addicted to them (without realising it), you may feel unwell, or even become quite ill with nausea, headaches, irritability and sleeplessness. Don't worry too much. These symptoms should not last more than four or five days. One week at the most. If they persist beyond that period, let your therapist or physician know urgently! Remember, giving up a favourite food can be just as bad as giving up a drug because the foods you are allergic to, or the foods that cause your illness, act just like a drug!

You can eat as much as you like, and as often as you like, provided you make your selections from this list. You should try to rotate the foods you eat, however, to minimise the possibility of becoming sensitised to a new food. Follow these guidelines:

1. Try not to eat the same food twice in any four-day period and certainly not twice on the same day.
2. Do not eat more than two to four single foods per meal; the less the better.

ILLNESSES ASSOCIATED WITH CFS

3   Avoid all junk foods such as lollies, cakes, pies, soft drinks, processed foods, colourings, etc.
4   Use sea salt whenever possible.
5   Use glass containers rather than plastic, and try to use distilled or filtered water.
6   Eat many small meals rather than a few large ones.
7   Herbal teas, nuts, tea leaves and any leftovers that may have mould growing on them (and they all do after 12 hours, although you can't see it) can be placed in a microwave oven for a few seconds. This will kill the fungi. An alternative is to place them on a white piece of paper and expose them to strong direct sunlight for a couple of hours.

Choose from these foods:

Vegetables   Apart from mushrooms, all fresh vegetables (except those you already know you are allergic to, if any) are permitted.
Fruit   Only avocado and a little freshly squeezed lemon, lime, or grapefruit juice are allowed.
Seeds and nuts   All seeds, fresh nuts and sesame butters are allowed.
Proteins   All fish, seafoods, poultry and meats are allowed. Although red meats are not recommended, some may be eaten in moderation. Turkey is the safest, followed by duck and lamb, then chicken, and then duck eggs or free-range chicken eggs. Pork and red meats should be eaten only as a last resort.
Fats   Only use olive oil for cooking and for salad dressings (with a few drops of lemon juice).
Fluids   Drink vegetable juices, mineral, soda and plain water (preferably filtered or distilled).
Carbohydrates   At this stage use only rice, millet, soya, lentil or potato flours. You can make yeast-free bread with them, or delicious pancakes to which you can add different flavours.
Foods to avoid   Remember: no alcohol, bread, pastry, pies, sweets, fruit, fruit juices or dried fruits. No milk, margarine, butter or cheese. Do not eat any processed foods, sauces, instant or packaged meals. No salad dressings or any foods that may contain yeast (see list on p. 161), grains, wheat flour or milk.

The MEVY (meat, eggs, vegetables and yoghurt) diet

This is another elimination diet which in many ways is the same as the diet we have just outlined. This diet also avoids most of the foods that commonly provoke allergic reactions. The guidelines and foods to eat are fairly similar to those of the elimination diet (see page 162), but there are some subtle differences:

1. Try not to eat the same food twice in one day if you are showing severe allergic reactions.
2. Do not eat more than two to four single foods per meal. If you have any food intolerances/allergies the fewer foods you eat the better.
3. Avoid all junk foods such as sweets, soft drinks, processed foods, preservatives, colourings, etc.
4. Use sea salt whenever possible.
5. Use glass containers rather than plastic, and try to use distilled or filtered water.
6. It is better to eat many small meals rather than a few large ones.
7. Herbal teas, nuts, tea leaves and any leftovers that may have mould growing on them should be placed in a microwave for a few seconds, or put on a piece of white paper in strong direct sunlight for a few hours.

Vegetables Apart from mushrooms all fresh vegetables (except those you may already be allergic to, if any) are permitted. Try to eat as many as possible raw. Please note that some individuals can be allergic to salycilates. If so, after suitable tests these should be eliminated

Fruit Only avocadoes and a little freshly squeezed lemon, lime or grapefruit juice are allowed

Seeds and nuts All seeds, fresh nuts and sesame butters are allowed

Proteins All fish, seafoods, poultry and meats are allowed. Although red meats are not recommended, some may be eaten in moderation. Turkey is safest, followed by duck, lamb, or lean beef, then free-range chickens and eggs. Pork and fatty red meats should be eaten only as a last resort!

Fats You should use olive oil for cooking and for salad dressings (with a few drops of lemon juice), but some linseed oil and fresh butter are allowed. No margarine!

Fluids Drink vegetable juices, mineral, soda and plain water — preferably distilled or filtered — and you can add some fresh lemon, grapefruit or lime juice for taste

Carbohydrates At this stage only use white rice, millet, soya, lentils and potatoes, or their flours. Some people can tolerate brown rice well, but others can't. It is best to avoid it for a few days, then add some brown rice to your diet to find out if you can tolerate it. You can make yeast-free breads with the flours listed above or delicious pancakes to which you can add different fillings

Foods to avoid Remember: no alcohol, breads, pastry, pies, sweets, fruit, fruit juices or dried fruit. No milk, margarine or cheese. Do not eat any processed foods, sauces, instant or packaged meals. Do not eat any salad dressings or foods that contain yeast (see p. 161), gluten grains (wheat, malt, barley or corn) and non-grain gluten substances (buckwheat, bananas or milk) because gluten can exacerbate fungal growth and irritate the intestinal tract. Gluten is a common allergen and while your immune system is under par you may become sensitised (allergic) to it, if you are not already.

Additional dietary information
- Cultured yoghurt should be eaten daily
- Seasoning and herbs are allowed
- Garlic should be used as soon as possible — ask your doctor
- Soya milk is allowed provided it does not contain malt or other grain additives
- Pure carob powder can be used
- Tomatoes are considered to be a vegetable, so can be eaten
- Tahini, cashew butter, chick peas, lima beans, tofu, and rice cakes and biscuits are allowed
- Brown rice is not allowed during the early stages; later you will be allowed to try it
- Sprouts, rye breads, goat's milk, skimmed milk, rolled oats, sesame oil, honey, tapioca, maple syrup, bean curd, chinese soy sauce, malt, dates and vegetable cooking oils are NOT allowed. Later these foods will be reintroduced to test your

tolerance of them. If in doubt you can be specifically tested for allergic responses to each food.

Making diets more interesting

If you are on a diet calculated to starve candida, or indeed on any elimination, low-carbohydrate, milk-free, yeast-free or grain-free diet, it might seem rather boring, but here is some help. With a little effort and by following the basic ideas given here you will learn what can be done with patience and imagination.

- Baked dinners are generally a good idea, provided you remember to use only olive oil for basting
- Salads are an excellent standby. To make them more interesting add some crab, chopped cold lamb, chicken (no skin) or turkey. Also try more exotic flavourings such as fennel
- Use this special salad dressing:
    1 tablespoon of olive oil
    juice from a quarter of a lemon
    some sea salt or celery salt and pepper
    Place everything in a small screwtop jar and shake vigorously
- Try stir-frying vegetables in a little olive oil, maybe adding some finely chopped parsley (and why not garlic, too!). You will be pleasantly surprised how different the vegetables can taste!
- Buy fresh minced lamb (cut off the fat before mincing) and some chicken (no skin) or turkey (it's less fatty and has a higher vitamin content than chicken) for a shepherd's pie, hamburgers or meat balls. Use only fresh tomato
- Experiment with various herbs but avoid mint, nutmeg, mace and chilli. Try fresh coriander, fennel or basil — they are great with salads
- Unfortunately eating out is, excuse the pun, OUT. Well, think of the money you'll save and all the old movies you can catch up with. Still, if you have to go out, stick to dry-grilled fish, salads without dressing (bring a little bottle of your own concoction), oysters or boiled prawns. When the dessert menu comes around, take a walk!
- If your friends invite you to dinner don't bore them with your problems, just tell them that you will BYO food. And do just

that, along with some distilled water, soda or mineral water and plenty of willpower. Of course if they are real friends, just send them a copy of this diet and they will prepare something adequate for you
- Don't forget your vitamins!

General guidelines for the treatment of systemic candidiasis

1   Accurate diagnosis will establish if candida is the *cause* of your problems or merely a *symptom* of another, perhaps more serious disease state.
2   Appropriate anti-fungal medications: these can be of different types, strength and dosage. Your therapist will decide which is most suitable for you. Please remember that while you may have heard that a medication is successful, it may not be successful for *you*.
3   Follow an appropriate anti-candida diet. Note that there are many of these diets, variously known as the elimination diet (see p. 162), candida control diet, mould avoidance diet, MEVY diet (see p. 164), etc. Although some, like the MEVY diet, seem to be the most useful generally, each diet may have to be specially tailored to your individual requirements. Again, remember that the diet that cured your best friend may not help you at all, and may even make you worse.
4   Avoid antibiotics, especially those of the broad-spectrum variety, unless absolutely necessary. Even then, take supplements and anti-fungals at the same time to minimise the side effects.
5   Discontinue the birth control pill if possible and avoid tampons.
6   Eliminate allergies as far as possible and avoid being exposed to allergens, especially moulds and fungi and their spores. Check your bedroom for airborne moulds. This can be done simply by obtaining special mould plates and for a nominal charge a mycologist will report in a few weeks on the type, number and species. Your therapist will then know if your environment is affecting you and, if you are allergic, arrange for desensitisation of the particular moulds you have been exposed to.
7   Take regular nutritional supplements calculated to prevent the growth and spread of candida.

8   Make sure you avoid sexual or intimate contact with people suffering from oral, vaginal or skin thrush.
9   Have regular tests before, during and after treatment to assess the seriousness of your condition and to monitor your progress and the efficacy of any treatment.
10 Be careful to practise the simple methods of hygiene outlined below.

Treating vaginal/genital thrush

The treatment of vaginal/genital thrush must include your sexual partner, too, to avoid reinfection.

Because, as we have already seen, vaginal or genital thrush is a localised infection of a candida problem that is already in the gut, you should take a course of prescribed anti-fungal treatment (such as pure Nystatin powder) and pessaries.

Make up the Nystatin solution as outlined on p. 159 and drink five tablespoons of it immediately after each dose of Nystatin powder. As I have already mentioned, the Nystatin solution can be used to swab infected ears, or gargled to treat the lower throat which often becomes a reservoir for candida organisms. The solution may also be used as a vaginal douche and should be used every night during treatment and, if possible, on awakening. After douching pure, cultured yoghurt can be applied directly to the vagina. Cover with a sanitary pad and leave overnight. Douche again on rising, or at least wash thoroughly. Use one pessary in the daytime only.

All sexual contact should be avoided for the first two weeks of treatment and any regular sex partner should be asked to take half a teaspoon of Nystatin powder twice daily with food for those two weeks only. Patients and their partners should also use the douche solution to swab their genital area after each bowel movement. Women should learn to wipe backwards after bowel movements and wipe themselves downwards after urinating. Always remember to wash your hands thoroughly; when you get up in the morning wash your hands and clean your nails carefully.

Underwear should always be rinsed in *hot* water. Women should avoid using panty liners and any other items which will impede the flow of air and contribute to the creation of moist, sweaty conditions in which candida thrives. Such conditions not only bring back or aggravate the problem but interact with residual detergents, causing local irritations which help the growth of more organisms. The use of tampons is not recommended. Depending on the material it is made from, underwear can be sterilised of candida by placing it in a microwave oven.

If you suffer from any degree of genital itchiness, inflammation or irritation a topical cream (such as Vaginol), which has tea-tree oil as an active ingredient, is to be recommended. Other substances which are beneficial are aloe vera and garlic.

Men may suffer from post-coital irritation or rectal/anal itching and frequently show symptoms such as groin skin rashes or tinea. In such cases it is essential they practise the hygiene measures outlined above and, in addition, apply anti-fungal creams to affected areas.

Once vaginal/genital thrush has been treated, it is important to prevent recurrence. Four steps must be taken to ensure this:

1. As I have already explained, your sex partner must be treated, and sexual contact should be avoided during the first two weeks of treatment. Both you and your sex partner must follow the hygiene methods described above.
2. You must continue treatment until tests show that the problem has been resolved, even if the symptoms abate earlier.
3. You must take preventative measures such as avoiding high sugar foods, taking regular probiotics, etc.
4. You must treat any underlying condition or factor that reduces your resistance (immunity) in general.

APICHS — Another Form of CFS?

APICHS is the acronym for Autoimmune, Polyendocrinopathy, Immune Dysregulation, Candidiasis, Hypersensitivity Syndrome.

In plain language it means a syndrome which involves:

- an overactive immune system;
- symptoms affecting most, if not all, of the endocrine glands;
- a badly regulated immune response;

- systemic and usually chronic candida infections (with or without manifest thrush);
- allergies.

As you can see, it would be quite difficult for the inexperienced diagnostician to differentiate between such a picture and one that is often accepted as that of CFS. APICHS sufferers have multiple allergies and symptoms that involve many organ systems. Many suffer with severe Pre-Menstrual Syndrome, some have thyroid malfunctions, respiratory allergies (sinus, asthma, post-nasal drip, mucus, hay fever, etc.). Blood tests often show immune abnormalities (T cell ratios). Skin tests for allergies turn out to be positive.

The scientists who named this condition were Phillip L. Saifer and Nathan Becker in the book *Food Allergies* (by Jonathan Brostoff and Stephen Challacombe). They suggest that much evidence exists for the fact that the environmental chemicals (xenobiotics) may trigger an overproduction of antibodies to specific organs. Such antibodies may also react with hormones or their receptors, as well as the gland that produces those hormones.

It is easy to see that such a state of affairs may well result in an illness or series of illnesses which can be mistaken for hormonal, or endocrinal, malfunctions. Which of course, they are, in a way.

Saifer and Becker believe many APICHS sufferers have a form of thyroiditis (inflammation of the thyroid) and list the following symptoms:

- morning tiredness;
- loss of short-term memory;
- asthma or other allergies;
- difficulty controlling weight;
- depression and other mood disturbances;
- emotional and psychological problems;
- bladder disorders such as increased frequency or urgency;
- changes in the ability to tolerate temperature changes; and
- menstrual irregularities.

As in all syndromes, please do not feel that if you have a few of these symptoms you are an APICHS sufferer. On the other hand, again as in all syndromes, it is possible to have APICHS and not experience all of the symptoms listed. Patients in this group often also suffer the symptoms of sinusitis, hives, eczema, headaches, irritable bowel, muscular pains and aches, arthritis-like joint pains and many food, chemical and drug intolerances.

DIAGNOSING APICHS

There are some subtle differences between APICHS and CFS sufferers. One of these is the fact that although both suffer with overwhelming fatigue, with APICHS the tiredness is often worse on awakening and lifts somewhat by late afternoon, when the adrenals are most active. This is not surprising, since the adrenals make some of the most important stress hormones. Interestingly, Chinese doctors have known this for a few thousand years and all acupuncturists are familiar with the 'Chinese clock' which shows adrenal functions and stress capacity increase between 4 pm and 6 pm. Who was it that said science tends to re-invent the wheel every few years?

Unfortunately, APICHS sufferers pay for this increase in energy by experiencing insomnia, disturbed sleep and headaches later in the night.

They often complain of feeling cold easily and are prostrated by hot days. They tend to be pallid, puffy and look pasty (the three Ps of allergic thyroiditis). Often there is a familial history of thyroid problems, allergies or autoimmune disease.

Victims are usually in their early twenties or forties and have a childhood history of ear infections, sore throats, recurrent antibiotics administration, skin rashes, eczema, digestive problems and sinusitis, hay fever or asthma. The problems are usually worse through adolescence when females often experience recurrent vaginal thrush. They are usually moody people who need a lot of sleep. Women suffer with periods of depression, especially likely to occur after childbirth. Many women develop cystic breasts (non-malignant lumps), endometriosis and even mitral valve prolapse (a heart valve condition).

By the forties many have developed uncontrollable allergies and feel like they are falling apart. They become so sensitive they can't stand some perfumes, pesticides, car fumes, cigarette smoke and often alcohol. They tend to develop itchy skin or genitals and, if asthmatics, find they have to increase the frequency of medications. Muscles ache, vaginal thrush occurs and life becomes more and more unpleasant.

Such patients need their thyroid functions looked at very thoroughly and that means a lot more than just a thyroid function test. Apart from basal temperature readings, such patients need their anti-thyroid antibodies (anti-thyroid microsomal antibodies) and anti-thyroglobulin measured by RIA, not agglutination.

Thyroid medications are used, either homeopathic or herbal, with vitamins, minerals and selected amino acids, or patients are given hormone therapy. Depending on the stage of thyroid function, diets are prescribed that are free of factors that affect thyroid functions (goitrogens).

After investigating candida antibodies, one starts anti-fungal therapy, usually with nystatin powder, and then the candida antibodies are measured again to monitor progress.

Skin tests for allergies, followed by intradermal end pointing, allow the therapist to prepare suitable vaccines for the allergies and, together with counselling on avoidance techniques, this can be very beneficial. In some cases the allergies may need to be managed by more complex techniques to neutralise the allergies (such as intradermal titration).

In their conclusion, Saifer and Becker had this to say:

> Management of environment allergens is much more likely to be beneficial if concomitant autoallergy is effectively treated. The full spectrum of antigens to be considered must include candida and other 'normal' flora. The patient response to this comprehensive approach is often remarkable.

Depression and CFS

Depression is one of the most common symptoms of CFS. For various reasons it seems to affect a disproportionate number of females. Yet depression can be an illness in its own right.

Irrespective of whether it is a symptom or a clinical condition, there are many ways to help depressed individuals.

There are many types of depression and each one of them can have different causes.

Among them, although you might not believe it, are the lack of cuddles and of daylight. Missing out on these two things may not only cause depression — it can make you fat.

Often described as the common cold of psychiatry, depression is such a common problem that it is a rare human being who does not suffer from it at one time or another. When a psychiatrist speaks of depression, however, he or she is describing something clinical, or an illness of which there are many types. Each kind of depression can have several symptoms. After analysing the presenting symptoms a diagnosis of depression may be made. The type of depression diagnosed will depend on the symptoms, an analysis of the patient's history and perhaps some psychological or laboratory tests. Then, a suitable treatment is prescribed. It sounds quite simple. Alas! Simple it is not!

To start with many people who suffer from depression are also overweight. The therapist must always try to assess if any particular individual is depressed *because* he or she is overweight — or the other way around. The fact is that the two seem to go hand-in-hand in a considerable proportion of sufferers. Special assessment tests like the HOD (Hoffer and Osmond Diagnostic test) cards-sorting test are admirably suited to ferret out true clinical depression.

Another problem is that there are so many *kinds* of depression.

Depression can be unipolar ('simple') or bipolar. The latter is also known as 'manic depression' and a variation of it goes by the acronym of MDP, which is an acronym for 'manic depressive psychosis'. Then there is a variant known as SADS (for Seasonal Affective Disorders Syndrome). There is also PPD (post partum depression), as well as 'endogenous depression' (from within or spontaneous) and 'reactive depression'. This last one means you are depressed because that is the way you react to something or another that has happened to you.

Although endless lists of such causes of reactive depression can be, and indeed are, regularly compiled by learned psychologists, the fact is that some things affect some people more than others. One may become depressed by alcohol, sickness, the loss of a job, divorce or an unyielding mother-in-law. Some of us seem to shrug off adverse events like the proverbial water off a duck's back while others become depressed every time things don't run smoothly.

Given the infinite variety of humans, this is entirely understandable. It is only when an individual fails to recover after the causative event has passed, that such a permanently depressed state becomes a clinical illness.

Psychiatric medicalese is a veritable minefield of acronyms and a trap for the unskilled in semantics. The truth of the matter is that depression can be caused by almost anything: lowered immune responses, candida, alcohol abuse or over-indulgence, vitamin B12 deficiency, an imbalance or deficiency of several minerals, nutrients and amino acids, as well as different kinds of anaemia, malabsorption, hypoglycaemia and food allergies. APICHS (see page 169) causes a type of depression which can often be successfully treated by stimulating the thyroid and adrenal glands.

Depressed people can become obsessive or indolent; lackadaisical or compulsive; lazy or workaholics. In fact the full spectrum of possible individual reactions to depression is almost as varied as human nature. The only thing they have in common is depression. There are of course some well understood causes for depression. One can, for example, become depressed because of continuous or excessive stress. Nowadays we know that stress in general can cause the body's levels of noradrenaline (also called norepinephrine) to become exhausted. Low levels of noradrenaline are associated with depression. Treatment of individuals suffering this problem with drugs other than those elevating noradrenaline will not help alleviate the problem. Therapists familiar with orthomolecular (nutritional) psychiatry know only too well that otherwise useful nutrients like vitamin B6, tryptophan, zinc and high complex carbohydrates diets like vegetarianism or Pritikin will usually not resolve this type of depression and may, in some cases, make it worse.

Conversely, we know that whenever stress plays a strong contributing role in clinical depression, tyrosine is probably the treatment of choice. Depression often, but not always, goes hand-in-hand with low blood pressure, low blood sugar and low thyroid functions (all of which tend to keep one fat), as well as depleted adrenals. Tyrosine can normalise blood pressure, stimulate the thyroid and contribute to blood sugar stabilisation via adrenal support. Patients suffering with this kind of depression often crave a multitude of foods and, while these may include sweets, there often is a strong desire for cheese, chocolate and other tyramine-containing foods.

If digestion is impaired (as in low hydrochloric acid states or intestinal candidiasis for example) then dietary tyrosine will be converted to tyramine which in turn tends to stimulate the adrenals and cause further depletion of noradrenaline stores while at the same time depriving glands like the thyroid of needed tyrosine.

But just in case you think tyrosine is perfect, let me inform you that tyrosine, as indeed most aromatic amino acids, may be contraindicated in some types of schizophrenia. Orthomolecular practitioners are well aware of the contraindication of each amino acid supplementation in psychosis and usually assess patients very carefully before administering megadoses.

Lay readers are urged NOT to take large amounts of single amino acids if there is a history of mental illness, unless under the direction and supervision of a competent orthomolecular nutritionist familiar with this type of orthomolecular psychiatry (also known as precursors therapy). On the other hand, most of the beneficial effects of tyrosine, or the side effects of an overdose, can be wiped out by the simultaneous administration of large neutral amino acids such as valine. Caffeine tends to lower plasma levels of tyrosine and could therefore increase the effects of stress in general.

Certain forms of cancer, like malignant melanomas and glioblastoma multiforme, are known to soak up tyrosine at a great rate in vitro. It would be prudent therefore not to use this amino acid under such circumstances unless the possible advantages clearly outweighed the potential risks.

Of course there are some types of depression which respond poorly, or not at all, to tyrosine and need tryptophan instead. I clearly remember lecturing on the biochemistry of this problem (tyrosine vs tryptophan) back in 1974. It has taken almost fifteen years for this information to reach the popular literature. The clues to non-tyrosine-dependent depression are quite simple. Sufferers will almost invariably crave sweets and consume carbohydrates (complex or otherwise) at every opportunity. They may not do so at regular mealtimes but whenever they feel hungry, and this is usually mid-afternoon and late evening, they will choose carbohydrates. They will often have gigantic sandwiches at ungodly hours. If questioned, they admit that the actual filling is unimportant. As long as there is bread! As a general rule these depressed patients tend to have sleeping problems and usually respond well to tryptophan, another amino acid which can cross into the brain. Like tyrosine, tryptophan also comes from proteins but, unlike tyrosine, it requires the simultaneous presence of carbohydrates in order to enter the brain. Tryptophan is then changed into serotonin which is a neurotransmitter that can lift some types of depression, induce drowsiness and stimulate immune functions.

Bulimia is an eating disorder which causes sufferers to overeat, then purge themselves (induce vomiting) to keep their weight down. Many bulimics are also depressed. Interestingly, the same combination of carbohydrate cravings and depression is also found in several types of Pre Menstrual Syndrome. Many cases respond well to oral supplementation with tryptophan which also helps to reduce carbohydrates cravings.

LIGHT

While most of the research on this subject has been conducted by Drs Richard and Judith Wurtman of the Massachusetts Institute of Technology (MIT), it was psychiatrist Norman Rosenthal at the United States National Institute of Mental Health who first looked specifically at patients suffering with SADS.

The key to understanding SADS lies in a little gland called the *pineal,* which is situated at the base of our brain. It has been called the 'seat of the soul' (by Déscartes) and more recently the 'gland for all seasons' (by *New Scientist).*

We now know that people who suffer the blues all winter but obtain a reprieve every spring, suffer with SADS, and the cause of their problems, as well as their yearly spontaneous recovery is linked to the pineal gland. Named because of its shape (a little like a pine cone) the pineal is smaller than an aspirin tablet and it is now recognised as the seat of our biological clock — the organ responsible for our daily rhythms (circadian), most animals' mating seasons as well as daily and seasonal changes in biochemical functions.

The pineal seems to adjust the whole physiology of animals (including humans!) to their environment. It does that because

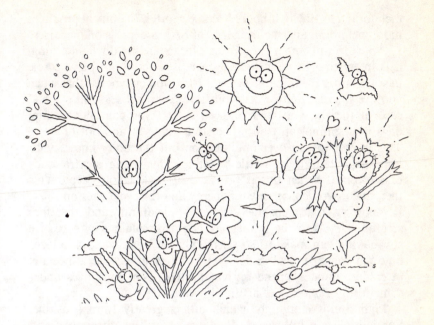

it is a 'neuroendocrinal transducer'. In other words it translates input signals such as light into nerve impulses which in turn stimulate endocrinal glands to produce a veritable cascade of hormones. These control, affect and modify almost all aspects of animal physiology, biochemistry and behaviour.

When light signals are scarce, or absent, the pineal activates two of its residing enzymes, NAT (N-acetyltransferase) and HIOMT (hydroxyindole-O-methyltransferase) which then begin to turn serotonin into the hormone melatonin. If you are susceptible, and SADS sufferers obviously are, the resulting lack of serotonin makes you depressed. Come spring and more daylight and the process is reversed. Hence the lift in mood.

In spite of the great importance of the pineal gland, it is not, as once believed, a master at all. It is, in fact, a slave under the control of yet another 'master clock' — the suprachiasmatic nuclei (SCN). This mass of specialised brain cells controls the pineal nightly output of NAT. Winter brings a definitive end of any mating urges animals may have and many animals tend to hibernate. It is now believed that the process is triggered by melatonin. As we have seen, the brain uses serotonin to make melatonin. As daylight hours become shorter, the pineal produces more melatonin and the incidence of SADS depression increases.

Apart from being a good reason for extending daylight saving, it is interesting to note that the increased serotonin plays a role in stimulating the immune system. Have you ever noted that when you are ill, especially when you have a viral disease like a bad case of the flu, you tend to sleep a lot? One can spend entire days in a somnolent, trance-like state going in and out of sleep. This is perhaps an oversimplification but the body knows your immune system needs a little boosting. This requires extra loads of serotonin. When this is provided, it makes you sleepy. This then makes you conserve your energy and the cycle goes on.

Knowing that sunshine decreases melatonin and therefore serotonin levels in the brain may help to explain why excessive sun baking can make us so sleepy while a brisk walk on a clear day can make us feel sexier. Yet millions of people, especially in colder climates, spend a great part of their daily lives under some form or another of artificial light.

Light bulbs emit light which differs greatly from sunshine. Sunlight casts a full range of colours as well as ultra-violet and infra-red. Incandescent light bulbs emit only the yellow, orange and red portion of the spectrum. Fluorescent lights work by passing a current through a tube of argon gas and mercury vapour. Thus 'excited' the mercury gives off a blueish light. This gives the characteristic 'cool white' we are all familiar with. Photobiologists are now finding that spending a lot of time exposed to only such 'cool white' portions of the light spectrum can upset the delicate human biochemistry in several ways by altering the ratio of hormones. It also can cause calcium malabsorption and deficiencies as well as a need for additional vitamin A. Unshielded fluorescent light may also add ultra-violet radiation so that sensitive people may become more susceptible to skin cancer.

Scientists are successfully treating SADS with high intensity light sessions. To produce the required effects one should use full-spectrum lights.

CHEMICALS AND DEPRESSION

Ask anyone what they think causes depression and you will hear many similar answers, such as: lack of money, overwork, unhappy relationships, stress — the list goes on. Ask a professional with a general knowledge of science and medicine, and the list will be the same, but with additional things like heredity, brain malfunctions or severe illness. Doctors or psychiatrists will then further add various complex brain chemicals (neurotransmitters) imbalances, childhood traumas and several diseases to that list. However, if you talk to an experienced doctor of environmental medicine (clinical ecology) or to an orthomolecular psychiatrist you will learn that depression can also be caused by allergies/intolerances to a variety of foods, inhalants and chemicals, as well as by nutritional imbalances or deficiencies that include vitamins, minerals and amino acids. As well you would be told that a variety of seemingly unrelated conditions, ranging from *Candida* infections to irritable bowel syndrome and latent viral re-activation can cause that mood disorder. Then you would also be told that long-term, low-grade exposure to xenobiotics (toxic, foreign chemicals), whether you are allergic to them or not, can also cause depression. Naturally, the same applies to short-term overexposure.

There are people who are unusually sensitive who, for one reason or another, react violently to a vast array of factors in their environment. The problem has been called PPS (Profound Sensitivity Syndrome).

While we all meet people who are *emotionally* very sensitive (the type that cries at the drop of a hat), there appears to be a certain proportion of the population which is very *physically* sensitive. And that does not just mean that they can't tolerate even the slightest pain. PPS individuals are usually creative, artistic, highly perceptive — and get their feelings hurt very easily. Some practitioners believe such individuals are more likely to suffer from autoimmune diseases such as lupus, MS (Multiple Sclerosis) or arthritis. According to American psychologist, Marc Lipton, such people are invariably right-brain dominant. Because such individuals perceive many events as stressful that others would consider trivial, they suffer the physical consequences of chronic, if low-grade stress. And environmental doctors have added a new dimension to this proposition. They argue, convincingly in my opinion and clinical experience, that people who are inherently emotionally hypersensitive are more likely to be susceptible to environmental pollutants in general, and xenobiotics in particular. There are already a number of physical illnesses, such as lupus, CFS, candidiasis and post-viral illness among others, whose manifestations include severe emotional disturbances. Often, in fact, such neuropsychiatric symptoms as depression, anxiety and paranoias are the first manifestations of some physical illnesses.

Whether because of heredity, past illness or life style, some people's nervous systems can be affected by exposure to viral or chemical agents. Usually, such damage manifests itself as mood swings, agitation, feeling spaced out, poor concentration and memory impairment — all signs of central nervous system depression.

Environmental illness specialists believe sensitivity to chemicals can be transmitted from mother to child. Dr William Rae, founder and director of the Environmental Health Center in Dallas, Texas, says:

> You can pass down chemicals and sensitivities from mother to child. It's seen in dope addicts and their babies, cigarette smokers and their babies and alcoholics and their babies. So it's not really startling that other chemicals are passed down. It's the logical extension. The data is there. If the mother had one part of styrene (a highly toxic xenobiotic compound which some plastic coffee cups and some insulation materials are made of) in her blood, the child may have two, or three parts in his.

As a result, such a child may be born with a predisposition towards profound sensitivity.

Dr Rae explains that conventional doctors and psychiatrists do not understand the interactions between environment and human beings. In his experience, a third of his depressed patients are in that state because they are exposed to chloroform. He has tested thousands of such patients and found high levels of that chemical in the blood of many. The situation is the same in Australia. For example chloroform is an anaesthetic and the steamy vapours which arise when you have a long, hot shower are full of it because of the high amount of chlorine in our household water. Now you know why a hot shower can be so relaxing and sleep inducing, while a cold one tends to be invigorating.

Interestingly though, depression, as well as other emotional problems, can also be caused by old viruses, which you may have contracted years, even decades, before without showing any symptoms at the time. When such viruses are re-activated years later, mood or emotional problems can occur.

Weight Problems and CFS

In the United Kingdom and the United States 33.5 per cent of the population are overweight enough to make the insurance man worry. In Australia it's about 20 per cent.

For years, obesity was approached by medical men in a simple, mechanical way — based on the old thermodynamic principle that energy cannot be created or destroyed. Hence, if x calories went in, and only half that amount came out in the form of heat and energy, then the other half must have turned into fat and you were plain greedy.

In the early 1970s, at the Department of Psychiatry at the University of Cincinnati, researchers fed same-size liquid meals to volunteers (some diluted and low calorie, some concentrated and therefore high in calories) and found that the next onset of hunger was related not to intake but to what each person *thought* he'd been given. More than adequately fed volunteers, believing they'd been given short rations, were physiologically hungry long before their colleagues who'd been short-changed calorie-wise, but who thought they'd had a fair share.

It's all it the mind!

The body, it's now known, has two systems for regulating food intake — a short-term one and long-term one. And the short-term day-to-day, hour-to-hour one, which is what we've been talking about above in the Schachter and Cincinnati trials, is not nearly as important as we've thought. As far as bodily housekeeping goes, it's the second system which, over months and years, regulates total body weight.

What this means is that the hypothalamus tends to look ahead and consider the overall situation, which is very wise of it from the point of view of survival. This seems to be why some animals can gorge in the summer and survive through the winter without fluctuating in weight.

The body, then, doesn't automatically make one extra kilo out of 7500 too many calories (or 31,500 too many kilojoules!) — the old equation — because the body can adjust its utilisation and metabolism according to input. That is, if less is eaten some people's metabolism is lowered and if more is eaten it is raised. This is why some lucky people who eat enormously don't put on weight, and unfortunates who start a slimming diet don't lose weight because their bodies cunningly arrange to get extra mileage out of what is being put in. (This must be how our ancestors survived periods of famine and hard winters, yet did not get fat in times of plenty.)

This process is known as thermogenesis, and although its efficient working appears to be largely inherited, correct early feeding in infancy and good habits like going for a walk after meals help to keep a good inheritance in shape. The old sick joke about exercise being no good because it takes ten hours of squash to get rid of 420 kilojoules (100 calories) is not really true. Regular exercise after meals does, long term, keep the thermogenesis working.

Obese people have faulty thermogenesis, and it is likely to get worse with age — though with age we also become lazier and usually greedier, or better able to indulge in large meals. Furthermore, it's better if you don't eat two large meals, but spread your intake over the day, because tests have shown that when a maintenance dose of kilojoules is given, people who consume it all in one go do put on weight.

The old cut-your-kilojoules-and-your-weight-will-cut-itself approach to weight loss is quite wrong. 'The average person,' says Dr John Yudkin, of *Sweet and Dangerous* fame, 'still believes overweight can be treated by diet in the same way as headache is treated by aspirin or appendicitis is treated by appendicectomy.' Which means the behavioural approach, of training yourself by aversion therapy or other forms of conditioning to just eat less, has big limitations. Weight is not a simple input/energy equation: there are other factors, from the interior.

Somewhere in there, in the hypothalamus or the brain generally, is the key. A further blow to the 'what goes in must come out as energy or go to your waistline' theory is that when students were fed between 4200 and 8400 (1000–2000 calories) extra kilojoules a day with a stomach pump, so that the brain knew nothing about it, they gained very little weight at all.

No matter your ancestry, you can still be started along the path to obesity at birth by the feeding practices of the Western world — namely, bottlefeeding and early introduction to solid food. The early months are the period when fat cells are formed for life, and in a well-stuffed baby fat cells are more abundant than in breastfed ones who are not prodded into early acquaintance with cereals and tinned dinners.

True, the obese child is not necessarily a fat adult. If you have willpower or luck on your side your extra fat cells will go through life in a deflated state and cause little trouble. Most fat babies, however, don't grow up to have willpower or luck on their side, and being overweight in infancy is an excellent preparation for being overweight in maturity. It is thought that poor nutrition and a high intake of carbohydrates at puberty, another growth period, make obesity more likely in maturity.

The biochemical changes underlying weight gain are where we begin to enter the territory of stress and allergy. And once we get away from the old idea that fat people, like alcoholics, are just short on willpower and 'moral fibre', the picture looks much more cheerful — or rather, your chances of doing something about it are rosier.

TYPE A EATERS
Dr H. Newbold, a psychiatrist and allergist and author of *Revolutionary New Discoveries About Weight Loss,* follows closely the idea of stress. There is the first reaction stage when a food tastes unpleasant; and the second addictive/adaptive stage which comes when we've persevered and learnt to like it.

Dr Newbold believes that just as there are two kinds of stress, before the third, ultimate stage when the whole show collapses, so there are two kinds of allergic weight people. The first type (type A) he calls the 'spree-eater'; and here, alas, it's not that one bite of the substance turns you off, but that it turns you on. And on and on, until you've eaten a whole chocolate cake or an entire plate of leftover lasagna, and would perhaps go out in the middle of a snowstorm to buy more, because you can't help yourself.

What happens, says Dr Newbold, is that our appetite control

centre in the brain (appestat) which normally tells us when to stop eating, simply doesn't swing into action. Experiments on the turn-on cells of the appestat show that when these are destroyed in experimental animals they just won't start eating and need force feeding. And experiments in mice, rats, cats, dogs, and monkeys show that when the turn-off cells are damaged or removed, there is no end to what can be shovelled in. In humans, doctors already know that some tranquillisers, like chlorpromazine, cause patients to overeat and grow excessively fat.

So, says Dr Newbold, there are substances, perhaps perfectly normal foods for some people, which in those who are susceptible go straight to the turn-off cells of the appestat — rather as pollen, in asthma sufferers, can go straight to the mucous membranes of the throat and nose. If people were obliging enough to die in the middle of an eating spree, says Dr Newbold, he's pretty sure that an autopsy would support his suspicions — that their turn-off cells were swollen, distorted and otherwise incapable of doing their job.

But while the outlook is rosy as regards tracking down offending foods which cause type As to behave like drug addicts (later I'll tell you how), detecting environmental substances which can also knock out your turn-off cells is harder. Did I say your environment is out to get you? Indeed it is! Here's a list of things Dr Newbold and many others have noted as affecting eating behaviour:

- Aftershave lotion
- Alcohol in any form (very common)
- Aluminium foil (the shiny side is coated with plastic)
- Anti-histamines
- Anti-perspirants
- Aspirin (which contains cornstarch, and other fillers)
- Cats (very common)
- Cockroaches
- Coffee
- Colouring and flavouring agents in soft drinks and low calorie drinks
- Chewing-gum
- Food colouring

- Fresh newsprint
- Fumes from city traffic
- Fumes from gas stoves
- Hot or cold weather, which may aggravate allergic reactions
- House dust
- Household cleaning products
- Room fresheners and deodorisers
- Insecticides
- Laxatives
- Lipstick
- Mould from plants, houses, cheese, yoghurt
- Paper cups and waxed cartons (which contain cornstarch)
- Perfume
- Plastics, especially soft ones
- Powder (cornstarch again)
- Tobacco (very, very common)
- Toothpaste
- Tranquillisers
- Vaginal creams, douches and foam
- Vitamins
- Water (chlorine, fluoride, mould)

With a list like this, and new substances are found to add to it every day, it's no wonder that a type A eater never knows the day or the hour when he/she'll be overcome with a compulsion. A visit to an office where they've just been painting, sharing a lift with a beautiful scented woman (or man), patting a passing cat, sniffing fumes from laboratories, kitchens or cars, even a harmless cup of coffee or a nap on the wrong kind of pillow can trigger it.

Holidays are a special hazard for the spree-eater —not so much the going abroad sort, which involves other bodily upheavals, but the good old traditional sort like Christmas. But although it's known that many people do get morose and wretched at Christmas, the standard explanation remains the psychological one: you're pining for your happy childhood, lost friends and relatives.

Children's birthday parties need special mention. Women who never have the slightest trouble resisting sweet goodies, but who can hardly knock back something offered by a smiling little child, may find that this sugary stuff — plus the necessary stiff drinks when the children are out of the way — brings on a classic and thunderous eating spree. Ordinary grown-up parties, where the food is largely unsugary and not artificially coloured, may prove harmless. Psychological explanations, that it's 'all emotional', that you can't, perhaps, accept that your little tot is growing up, are as suspect as the Christmas theory.

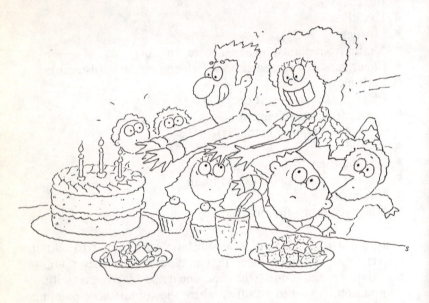

This, of course, points up the whole craziness of the way we feed our children — hopelessly hooking them almost from birth (especially premature babies who tend to be hypoglycaemic) on sugars and manufactured foods, so that they have to spend the rest of their lives nibbling celery sticks and avoiding the peanut bowl at parties.

Food colourings and chemicals: we've heard about these often from nutritionists and environmentally conscious people. But it is not often realised that they can trigger bouts of gluttony, and the awful loathing and depression that follow.

Tobacco, even other people's cigarette smoke, is already known to damage the lungs. But Professor Roger Williams, at the University of Texas, believes it can damage the appestat centre of the brain in some people; and Dr Newbold reports patients who become violently hungry after one cigarette — despite what we know about cigarettes curbing appetite. We're all different.

Cannabis is a great example of a substance that brings on a wild desire to eat, and especially to drink milk. People who enjoy pot are allergic to either or both.

Alcoholics, too, may sometimes be victims of allergy. Dr Abram Hoffer, the Canadian psychiatrist and orthomolecular nutritionist who treats patients with large doses of niacin and vitamin B6, has found that some alcoholics have no compulsion to drink once they can be persuaded to switch drinks; to have, say, vodka instead of bourbon. Because it's not the alcohol but the substance from which it's made they're allergic to. One of Dr Newbold's bourbon drinkers, with a long history of food allergy and being overweight, gradually lost interest in drinking after switching to Scotch whisky.

Dust sensitivity is also common in type As, and is more marked in cold weather, when weight watchers generally have more trouble. Keep the air humid, and reduce dust in your home by getting rid of as much drapery and upholstery as possible. Keep books under glass. Heating systems don't help, and an oil-treated fibreglass filter may help by catching dust more efficiently. Dust which settles on radiators and the fins of heating apparatus becomes carbonised, so that the small particles are literally fired and become lighter than before; hence they float in the air longer and you absorb them more through your lungs. Consider tiled floors or polished wood.

A product called Dust Seal can be applied not only to furniture and fabrics, blankets and carpets, but to your family pets once a month, anything else that's non-washable every five years.

After wading through this, you'll understand that eternal vigilance is necessary. Just make sure, if you're overweight, that you eat only simple, unprocessed foods: meat, fruit, vegetables, and other non-manufactured products that do not come from packets, tubes and tins. And it's best to remove lingering pesticides by washing anything you're not peeling in warm water and Ivory soap, or Rokeach, and then rinsing thoroughly. (Rokeach is a kosher soap, made in New Jersey and exported worldwide. In Australia, try Solomon's Kosher Soap. The nearest to Ivory is Sunlight.)

And don't forget that allergic reactions to the chlorine and fluorides in city drinking water are fairly common, and spring water may contain moulds and algae particles. So your best bet is to bring a large, uncovered pot of tap water to the boil. Immediately it starts to boil, remove it from the heat and place it on a cold surface, such as a sink. You will notice a white vapour escaping from the pot: much of the chlorine is removed. Do not allow the water to boil for any period of time as this will only concentrate many of the contaminating chemicals present. After cooling, pour the boiled water into bottles, half filled, and give them a good shake to get back air and give it a more normal taste.

TYPE B OBESITY

Type B obesity people don't rush about blindly in search of anything as long as it's sweet, or polish off anything and everything they can find in the refrigerator. Type B fatties know exactly what they want in life and, in fact, know that they just don't feel right without, say, an egg for breakfast or a chocolate mint after dinner.

And they are right — they don't! Because they are addicted, as sure as any drug addict. Life for type Bs just isn't right until they've had their coffee, or their bedtime milk, or their mid-morning doughnut. In the pure type B, the twitch, or craving comes on very punctually — at whatever time of day the fix is needed. They are restless and edgy immediately before, for the simple reason that it is now twenty-three hours and fifty odd minutes since the last fix and, did they but know it, they are experiencing withdrawal symptoms, like any junkie.

Many people are combination type A and type B fatties, that is, they're addicted and go on little binges. But in the pure type B addictive eaters sprees are unknown; in fact they may pride themselves on sticking to a regular, sensible diet and never going off the rails.

Of course, not all addictive eaters are obese. Some are fortunate enough to be addicted to something non-fattening, like orange juice, or tea, or coffee — although in excess even these can get you into other sorts of trouble.

Aren't addictive eaters more likely to be of the well-regulated, or even compulsive, type who want everything done just so, day after day? How does this type of allergy start? More importantly, why can't overweight people realise that the 'little of something sweet' after meals or the extra slice of toast at breakfast is what is making — and keeping — them fat? These are common attitudes and questions people ask.

The overweight, addictive eater, sad to say, is often the victim of other factors; and despite what I've said earlier about traditional 'psychological' explanations for Christmas depression, these psychological factors do exist and can work in a horrible harmony with physiological ones.

Many overweight people are depressed. They are short on hope. For some people, rolls of fat become a convenient alibi: they're not successful, rich and famous because they're fat; and if their doctor were magically to make them thin, and they were still unsuccessful, poor and obscure, how dreadful! So, better stay in behind that comforting, sheltering, cosy fat. But fat people aren't happy; and when you're feeling low nothing cheers you up like food.

It is now known that tiny particles of food can leak through the gut into the bloodstream, without being broken down; and in some susceptible people these tiny particles weasel their way into cells and become incorporated in the body's metabolic machinery, so that the whole body chemistry becomes dependent on a steady supply of this material. You can see, then, how at risk the allergic person is when he starts to nibble his way out of a depression.

Cheering up is all very nice, but it may soon happen that you need cheering up daily, perhaps long after the initial depressive phase has gone; and so addiction is born. It's thought that, in women, alcoholism often follows this pattern, particularly after major life changes like divorce, menopause, hysterectomy or mastectomy.

Because eating the food to which you have an allergic addiction makes you temporarily feel better, you can soon be firmly hooked into eating a little of it every day and being convinced that it is actually good for you. This is what psychologists call 'reinforcement', and you can see how, in no time at all, you pile on extra pounds if your addiction happens to be high in calories: worse still, the very thought of giving up something that makes life worth living is unthinkable.

There are two ways to tackle this: strengthen the body's resistance and track down the offending substance. Once an allergic obese patient is given the ideal vitamin and mineral, and perhaps hormonal, level for her/him, the body is much better able to handle these problem food particles. And after a complete avoidance of the suspect substance for anything from two weeks to a year, depending on the individual, the cell's overtaxed chemistry may be able to return to normal.

Experienced doctors have invariably found that patients who have a marked food allergy at the root of obesity suffer withdrawal symptoms such as nervousness, depression, confusion, anger, paranoid suspicions and physical troubles like vomiting, diarrhoea, sweating and weakness — not unlike morphine addicts undergoing the cold turkey stage. By the fourth day, these symptoms magically vanish.

And one of the major addictive substances, a drug, if you like, is sugar, the very thing that the human race just didn't have a chance to eat at all until the last century. Though we don't usually think of sugar as a drug, it can certainly fit very nicely into the characteristics used by the World Health Organisation to define drug addiction, namely, 'An overpowering desire or need to continue taking a substance; a tendency to increase the dose; a psychic or psychological, and sometimes a physical dependency on the effects of the drug.'

Here is a questionnaire to help you identify type B obesity. Often, being obese is defined as 9 kilograms (20 pounds) above the normal, but we think you should consider that you might be obese if you are more than 4.5 kilograms (10 pounds) over your ideal weight.

1. Do you often yearn for a particular food?
2. Do you feel dissatisfied unless you eat a certain food?
3. Do you feel any of these symptoms before eating: weakness, tiredness, headache, restlessness, depression, irritability?
4. Do the above symptoms disappear after you eat?
5. Do you daydream about a certain food?
6. Will you go out of your way to locate one certain food that you crave?
7. Do you stock up on some foods to make sure you always have a good supply?

8   Do you buy books on how to make certain food, for example, bread?
9   Do you feel dissatisfied unless you finish a meal with something sweet?
10 Are you famous among your friends for a certain recipe?
11 Do you use lots of chemicals as household cleaning aids?
12 Have you lived near an orchard or anywhere near agricultural spraying with pesticides?
13 Has your home been sprayed by chemical pest control?
14 Do you feel unwell or have food cravings after you have been exposed to chemicals or allergens.

If you answered Yes to five or more of these questions, start thinking about chemicals, allergy and addiction.

There's no hard and fast dividing line. You can be basically a type B fatty with interludes of type A binges — going mad every so often for, say, popcorn, and coasting along the rest of the time with your daily fix of soft drink or coffee laced with sugar. But even this can be dealt with.

It's possible to have either a fixed allergy or a cyclic allergy to a fattening food. Most doctors understand only the fixed type of allergy; but according to Rinkel, Randolph, and Zellerk, in *Food Allergy*, only 5 per cent of food allergies fit this category.

Cyclic food allergies, as the name suggests, come and go, the critical thing being how frequently you eat the problem food and how much you eat.

The basic trouble here is the enzyme. We inherit our enzymes, which are protein, vitamin and mineral mixtures, just as we inherit height and hair colour. Well, you may be unlucky enough to draw some pernickety enzymes, only able to function provided they get ideal nutrition and not too much harassment; liable to sulk if their environment is not perfect, that is, if they are subjected to a barrage of a substance that requires them to work overtime.

You may have an enzyme system that feels that eating pumpkin once a week is really enough — in which case you just may co-exist harmoniously with your twitchy enzyme all your life, unless you wind up in an institution where they're very keen on giving you pumpkin every second day. How often is too often? This is something you can find out pretty simply with tests I shall outline later.

In obesity allergy, though, the villain is more likely to be something containing carbohydrate in a rather more thrilling form than pumpkin. Say, something with sugar, or maybe nuts. But, sad to say, there's one food on the suspect list that most of us would unhesitatingly call the dieter's best friend: cabbage.

Low as it is in calories, and regardless of all its wonderful roughage, minerals and vitamins in the raw state, cabbage has one big drawback: it contains a factor that may slow down your thyroid and therefore the rate at which you burn or utilise your food.

Dr Hans Selye has recently been working on a newly discovered group of hormones called catatoxic steroids. These hormones stimulate the formation of enzymes that can destroy the toxic substances usually produced by a stress situation. Smoking, for instance, introduces toxic chemicals into the bloodstream. If catatoxic hormones, the goodies, are efficient, they can destroy nicotine and cancer-causing chemicals. But if the stress level is too high for too long they are powerless against the rising tide of toxicity in the body.

Furthermore, if cancer-causing chemicals are introduced into the body in food, water or air, the equilibrium is further disturbed and the risk of cancer increases.

In other studies, Dr Selye was able to induce arthritis, ulcers, heart disease and other disorders simply by subjecting test animals to stress. The bright side, however, is that animals can be taught to avoid stress situations; and if humans, too, can learn to handle stress the future looks brighter.

Unfortunately it's trickier for humans to avoid stress than it is for animals. Certainly we can follow the Alcoholics Anonymous advice about changing what can be changed in our lives, and accepting what can't, and — most crucial of all — learning to recognise which is which. But when it comes to food allergy, especially a masked allergy which masquerades as an addiction, this cannot be done without expert help.

With CFS patients it's a little bit more complicated.

If one's liver has been affected by a virus, this will tend to make the body detox system work less efficiently. Of course it can also happen because of drug taking, some medications, alcohol and a host of other reasons. The point is that once the body finds it difficult to get rid of unwanted chemical guests, it wants to shut them up in fat tissue and this creates the infamous 'spare tyre'!

The opposite is also possible. A naturally thin person may not be able to produce enough fat to store dangerous chemicals. Such an individual will be more easily affected by a small amount.

Some chemical exposure may be beyond our control, and we may not even know it happened — yet it can affect us.

But we do know that chemicals, viruses and other factors can make a person become 'allergic' to substances they have eaten all their lives with impunity. When that happens, chances are the allergenic foods, as they are called, may contribute to one's weight problem.

Treating Chronic Fatigue Syndrome

There are many different ways to treat CFS, as well as each one of the symptoms that manifest themselves as a result of the syndrome in different individuals. It is the same for most illnesses. With treatments ranging from chiropractic to surgery and from acupuncture to herbalism we all know, have seen, or have heard of 'miraculous cures' for everything from ingrown toenails to cancer.

The dilemmas facing both patients and doctors alike is always the same: what will work best? What will work for me? Will the treatment that helped another person help me? There are no easy answers to these questions but I will tell you a couple of stories that I hope will illustrate both the way doctors and therapists can help people, as well as the pitfalls we all face.

A long time ago I had a patient with a gall bladder problem. Try as I might, nothing would help. Diets, regimens, cleansing — all were to no avail. A few months later my patient came to me and asked me to cure her headaches. Curious, as I had not seen her for some time, I asked her about her gall bladder pains. 'Oh', she replied matter-of-factly, 'I went to a zone therapist (people who apply pressure to specific points, similar to acupuncture points, on the soles of the feet). She asked me to take my shoes off, pressed a bit here and there, and the next day the pain was gone.'

The next time I had a patient with a similar problem I referred him to a zone therapist. It was no help at all! I then placed the patient on a special diet and the problem disappeared.

The moral of the story? Different people will be helped by different methods; no system is inherently better than another. It is people who are different — every person is biologically individual, as I have already explained. It is so important to remember this when prescribing treatment. Certainly some treatments work more often than others, but no treatment will work on every patient in every case.

Whether you are a patient, a doctor or a therapist, NEVER get stuck in the rut of using just one treatment, one routine, one method, one diagnosis ... Never assume that your piece of the puzzle is bigger and better or more important than the other pieces. The only one that counts is the *last* piece: the one that gives you the final and complete picture. Often it is only by finding the last piece that you can solve the mystery. And often it is not you that has the missing piece but someone else.

A few examples will make this clear:

SUPPLEMENTS
Therapists sometimes advise patients to take this or that vitamin, for example, a vitamin C powder with bioflavanoids. And for good reason, as bioflavanoids will enhance the absorption of vitamin C as well as provide additional health benefits.

Unfortunately some people are allergic to bioflavanoids. Salycilate intolerant individuals can become quite ill when taking such supplements. It may cause them to switch off the therapy, may aggravate allergies, or slow down progress. Or, at best, any advantages accrued by the vitamin C and bioflavanoids will be wiped out by the allergy/intolerance to that substance.

All this can also happen with the different forms of minerals, amino acids, herbal preparations and so on. I have seen people who can tolerate a particular supplement only in *one brand*. Perhaps the preparation methods or the fillers used do not agree with some. There are many forms of vitamins, minerals and other supplements. One person may tolerate, for example, a yeast-based selenium; another might only be able to take it in its sodium selenite form.

DIETS
The same thing applies to diets. Some vegan diets are counterproductive in cases of chemical overloading. Sometimes

it is necessary to *increase* cholesterol levels a little. Sometimes it is necessary to avoid all fruit, or only those high in natural salycilates. At other times it may be important to avoid those vegetables that affect the thyroid.

Some people should not have grains, whole or otherwise, while, occasionally one finds individuals who can eat white, refined bread but are severely affected by wholegrain breads. Some people can tolerate some grains, but not others. Occasionally we see people who cannot tolerate even rice.

As we have learned, the liver is central to any process of detoxification as well as immune system recovery. Yet the liver is the only organ that derives its energy not from blood sugar but from the constituents of proteins — amino acids. Yet the liver has to work to break food down into the amino acids (it is a process called deamination), and this creates another dilemma. If you do not get enough high quality proteins, the liver may not be able to do its job. On the other hand, it may be already in such a state that the additional work of obtaining the amino acids from foods is too much. So one will find that it is sometimes necessary to prescribe a high protein diet, but at other times a low protein diet. Even then the *type* of protein may make all the difference. Egg yolks, for example, contain all sorts of factors, including a type of phospholipid that actually helps the body fight viruses and the liver to take care of foreign chemicals.

Polyunsaturated fatty acids (found in some vegetable oils) are excellent and often needed. Some are essential. Yet certain fatty acids from some common oils have been shown to accelerate the growth of pre-existing tumors. Others, or an incorrect ration of them, can make inflammation more difficult to treat. Chemically overloaded people attempting detoxification may have problems if they eat lots of polyunsaturates for the simple reason that these oxidate and produce free radicals.

OXYGEN THERAPIES

Ozone is an oxygen with three atoms of oxygen rather than two. What this means is that the oxygen is activated. Pure oxygen with a high electrical discharge from a generator produces medical ozone. It tends to support the liver's efforts at detoxification and improves the metabolism of cells markedly, making them better able to provide more energy for the whole body. It improves circulation and reduces the clotting of red blood cells, thus improving their capacity to transport oxygen to where it is needed in the body. It also kills many species of bacteria, viruses and fungi. It is said to have the ability to revitalise, rejuvenate and regenerate body functions. For what it's worth, it is one of singer Michael Jackson's favourite treatments. If you've ever seen him dance you'll see why I mention this!

Mark Florence, one of the world's leading experts on oxygen, free radicals, etc., told me that oxygen therapies may well be a new way of approaching some diseases, but he reminds us that one must always remember that by using compounds like hydrogen peroxide in oxygen therapy you are employing one of the most potent toxins in nature. We have to find the dose that is low enough not to cause harm, but high enough to be useful. The trouble is that we don't know what the right dose is yet. Knowing this, my advice is *never* try some of these therapies without the consent and supervision of an experienced medical practitioner, preferably an environmental medicine specialist.

INTRAVENOUS VITAMIN C THERAPY

In my clinical experience intravenous vitamin C (IVC) is the single most helpful procedure for treating CFS patients. Very few people fail to respond at all, although the degree of response can vary greatly and the time it takes to work also covers a wide range.

I believe that the main problem with IVC is that everything about its administration must be personally tailored to each individual case. How much, how often, with which fluid, what to add to the vitamin C infusion (whether it is calcium, magnesium, zinc, vitamin B6, amino acids or trace elements) all must be carefully considered to obtain the best results. What the patient takes orally before the procedures may also be very important. We find some people need to be loaded up for a few days, as it were, with all sorts of adaptogenic factors, such as Siberian ginseng. In others it may not be as important or even necessary. In *all* cases, however, it is very important that one keeps on taking high doses of *oral* vitamin C powder before, during and for a while after the IVC procedure. In fact, the best way to determine the efficacy of IVC is for the patient to carry out a bowel tolerance procedure before and during IVC treatment.

The procedure is as follows: take a teaspoon of vitamin C powder (preferably with a compound of other factors but *not* calcium ascorbate or an alkaline formula: we use Viro C) every hour until you experience diarrhoea (let's say eight teaspoons evenly spaced during a day). Note the number of teaspoons needed to provoke this response. Next day take a little less than that number of teaspoons (in this example, say, six or seven). Reduce the intake gradually to the amount that you can tolerate. When you experience diarrhoea on taking four or five teaspoons per day, the IVC has probably achieved its maximum effect.

Naturally this procedure, known as the cathcart bowel tolerance method, cannot be used by everyone as some people will, for a variety of reasons, be unable to take sufficient vitamin C powder. If they suffer, for example, from gastric problems, an irritated stomach, etc., they would experience diarrhoea at a very small dose. In such cases IVC must be given without taking the additional oral vitamin C powder.

There are few and generally transient side effects to IVC, which is as safe as any such procedure can be. Some symptoms, like a sore throat, glandular swelling, headaches, feeling hot, mild sweating — all rather like having a mild case of the flu — are actually positive symptoms that we try to stimulate. Again, an experienced therapist knows when the symptoms are positive and when they may be a warning signal, which will lead them to vary the treatment procedures accordingly.

Response to procedures

The response to any procedure can vary enormously from person to person. I have seen people who benefit from small infusions of intravenous vitamin C. Others will only get better if the dose is much greater. The same applies to frequency.

People can benefit from ozone or hydrogen peroxide therapy. Others will not be touched by it and some can get worse. The list is endless, so please do not expect to find a one shot method of curing *anything*, let alone something as complex as Chronic Fatigue Syndrome.

You should learn all the possible ways in which you may be helped and all the different techniques that may work on you. Never assume that because something helped a friend it is therefore guaranteed to be the answer for you.

A good diagnostician and a good therapist will have at least some ideas about the course of treatment he or she will chart for you. And then will be flexible enough to alter the program as time goes by. Plotting a course of treatment is just like navigating a ship through a storm in an uncharted area that has rocks everywhere, of which you can only catch the occasional glimpse.

Treating CFS is just like navigating a ship in treacherous conditions. The therapist is the captain and he must rely all the time on the shouts of the patient who, after all, is measuring the waters with his or her own feelings.

Another point. Sometimes a test, a procedure, a diet or some other form of diagnosis will show only one small, seemingly insignificant deviation from normal. Usually it means just that. But sometimes it is like seeing an iceberg on the horizon. It may mean that, like an iceberg, what one sees is but a small portion of what lies underneath. Hidden, but deadly. An example of this arises when testing for allergies. Sometimes we see people who have no positive reactions whatsoever, except for a slight weal response to a single chemical. The textbook says this is of no consequence. And most times the book is right. But most books on the subject were written many years before the current xenobiotic explosion had taken its toll. Often we find such responses suggest that a particular individual is in fact allergic, overloaded or hypersensitive to many chemicals. But such sensitivities are buried under the surface. Unseen but dangerous. Just like the iceberg.

Finally, remember that when something fails, it is worth trying something else. There are so many ways to help your body fight it would be impossible to list them all or to be able to choose the method that is immediately right for you. I have seen many cases where after trying all the methods we were familiar with without much success, the patient has turned to a form of treatment that would appear to have no relevance. Yet in some cases this new treatment works.

As Mark Donohoe says, the 'last anchor' may well be a diet, a vitamin, a therapy, psychological counselling, a change of mental attitude, osteopathic or chiropractic manipulation, acupuncture, hydrotherapy, a further change in lifestyle, meditation ... the list of possibilities is endless. Sometimes the last anchor is pulled up by pure serendipity, as the following case history demonstrates.

Phyllis was a CFS patient. She was also very allergic, had a latent virus problem (Epstein-Barr and CMV) and a chronic candida infection.

Treatment was progressing well and Phyllis was improving — but not enough. She was allergic to wheat (a gluten grain), so I had placed her on a gluten (wheat, rye, barley, malt, buckwheat) avoidance diet. She was allowed to eat rice, millet and corn, which do not contain gluten. All the tests showed that she was not allergic to non-gluten grains and even challenging her with them provoked no reaction.

One day a friend gave her a pendulum and showed her how to use it to identify foods or other substances which may affect her. To her amazement when she swung the pendulum over a bowl of white rice (you have to actually hold the substance in your hand before you do this) it indicated that rice was not good for her. She stopped eating rice. From that day she improved.

Was the rice the last anchor? Was the pendulum the straw that *saved* the camel's back? Sometimes patients do this with their vitamins and discover that some affect them negatively. When they change the type, the brand or the formula, things get better.

Having said that, and continuing to keep it in mind, there are some basic principles about treating CFS holistically that have a general application:

1. You need an accurate diagnosis after a thorough interview and test routine.
2. Any serious underlying condition (diabetes, heart disease, cancer, etc.) obviously must be treated.
3. All symptoms, triggering and aggravating factors must be investigated and treated.
4. The twin principles of biochemical individuality and total load must be respected as far as possible.
5. Your lifestyle, diet, environment, etc., must be made as healthy as possible.
6. Anything that is stressful must be removed or reduced and everything possible must be done to increase the body's own fighting ability.

7   If any symptoms turn out to have a separate identity or cause then they must be taken care of. Examples are candida, LIAS, intestinal dysiosis, parasites and anaemias.
8   Allergies/intolerances must be investigated and taken care of. As I explain in other parts of this book, there are many ways to test, desensitise, neutralise and avoid all allergies. Each individual has to be assessed for the most suitable techniques for them.
9   Check for the possibility of chemical exposure, overloading, hypersensitivity and other environmental factors such as 'sick building syndrome', chemical outgassings in your home, sensitivity to electromagnetic radiation, toxic dental amalgam (mercury), etc.
10 Correct any nutritional imbalances or deficiencies that may exist. This is easier said than done, but please consider the fact that one may not be deficient in anything yet suffer from an *imbalance*. Plenty of copper and enough zinc may, however, unbalance the copper to zinc ratio and cause problems in some individuals. Then there are other nutritional factors such as essential fatty acids, amino acids, etc., that can cause problems when they are unbalanced in an individual.
11 Begin a process of detoxification and help your body, especially your liver and digestive tract, do its own elimination. This will vary greatly. For example, exercising to the point of sweating will often help chemically overloaded individuals but will make viral victims much worse. Chemical patients will benefit from saunas but should only take them for very short periods of time at first. Viral CFS sufferers can benefit from long, repeated saunas much sooner. Niacin flushing is very helpful in detoxification procedures. Some allergic people can't and should not use this method which may cause other problems.
12 Evaluate *all* other possible therapies.
13 Avoid pharmaceutical drugs unless absolutely necessary and even then take precautions if possible.
14 Generally speaking try to use foods and liquids that are as free of pollutants, additives, colourings, chemicals, etc., as possible. CFS sufferers should only drink filtered, distilled

or pure water (from glass containers) and obtain as much free-range and organically grown food as possible.

15 Alcohol is always contraindicated because it affects the liver and it shares some of the natural liver detox pathways with toxic chemicals. Alcohol will tend to slow down the process and may overload the needed pathways.

16 Vitamin injections are often very useful, at least in the early stages and when absorption problems are suspected. However, please note once again that what will help one person may not benefit another. For example, some vitamin injections contain niacin or nicotinamide (two forms of vitamin B3) and these can cause reactions in susceptible individuals. Other formulas contain lots of folic acid, a necessary and very useful nutrient. But some women who have pre-menstrual problems or suffer from endometriosis or pelvic inflammatory disease (PID) are either unusually sensitive to oestrogen (the female sex hormone) or their liver is unable to reduce the blood oestrogen levels after it has completed its mission, and because folic acid is synergistic with oestrogen, one occasionally encounters patients who will suffer needlessly when folic acid is given intramuscularly or intravenously. Some people are so sensitive in fact, that even a diet high in some vegetables which contain factors that interact with oestrogen (the so-called phytoestrogens) may aggravate their symptoms. This can sometimes happen to women with poor thyroid functions.

Immune boosting supplements abound. Echinacea is one of the best but very high doses (more than 20 of the common capsules a day) may achieve the opposite effect. The same applies to vitamin E and to zinc, which reduce the efficacy of our immune system if taken in doses that are too high.

Glycyrrhiza (from licorice) is to be avoided by patients with kidney problems or by those whose adrenal glands produce excessive amounts of certain hormones. Glycyrrhiza may cause the body to retain excessive fluid and some anxious patients may become worse. The Japanese mushroom extract marketed as Reishitaki or Rehishigen powder (also known as LEM, from *Lentinus endodes*, an immature form of the shiitake mushroom) appears to have both an immune boosting and antiviral effect. With some CFS patients it works almost miraculously. With others the cofactor Q10 produces similar results. Some people need both.

17 The *timing* of supplements and medications may be very important. Directions like 'take three times daily' may not be good enough. Viral CFS patients should take magnesium in the morning and calcium at bedtime and *never* take calcium in the form of calcium lactate.

It is doubtful if calcium supplements are useful for chemically sensitive people, yet the absorption of some specific dangerous substances is inhibited by calcium.

Tyrosine, an amino acid often prescribed to stimulate thyroid functions, to overcome stress, to curb appetite, ameliorate depression and help immunity, is often only useful if taken early in the morning on an empty stomach.

Garlic is an excellent natural antibiotic, antioxidant, anti-candida product, etc. However, according to some researchers it can be counterproductive during the early stages of the treatment of intestinal candida infection because it may drive the candida into recesses of the gut from where it may be even more difficult to eradicate them.

Vitamin B5 (pantothenic acid) can aggravate anxiety states in susceptible individuals, and late in 1990 we learnt that both biotin and cysteine will actually promote the growth of candida organisms. We stopped using them in those circumstances and noted the difference.

18 Candida infections and allergies must be taken care of. Homeopathic measures will generally not help severe candida cases which need specific anti-fungals, but will often help allergic and chemically overloaded or immunodeficient people. Those who are chemically sensitive sometimes do better with homeopathic allergy treatments with or without desensitising techniques.

19 Most patients need adaptagenics (tonics) such as ginseng, as well as specially tailored supplement regimens. But Korean and Siberian ginsengs are quite different. For some people only one works, while the other causes problems.

20 Always remember that CFS treatment can take weeks, sometimes months to achieve results but if the patient relapses or is not improved, the physician should look for other causes or contributing factors.

To summarise — some of the more successful treatment regimens for CFS are:

- a diet appropriate to the patient's allergies, intolerances and hypersensitivities after suitable testing, as well as specific nutritional requirements
- the use of specific supplements/nutrients targeted at the basic underlying problem and the corollary symptoms. In general these will include shiitaki, echinacea, vitamin C, co-factor Q10, primrose oil for viral problems and antioxidants/amino acids for chemically induced CFS
- gamma globulin for viral/liver involvement with perhaps intravenous vitamin C or oxygen therapies (intravenous hydrogen peroxide or ozone)
- detoxification manouevres such as niacin and saunas for chemical CFS
- fasting and challenges for some types of allergies. Environmental control for others. In some cases desensitising sublingual vaccines (drops) are very useful, but at other times serial dilution neutralisation may be necessary. Homeopathic liver, immune and allergy preparations are often used and sometimes the effect of these is assessed against that of other therapies to see what is most suitable.

In my experience, most CFS sufferers can be improved considerably within two or three months. Sometimes it takes longer, and in such cases there are always a multitude of other contributing factors, whether physical or emotional, that slow down the progress or recovery.

THERE ARE NO PROBLEMS IN MEDICINE — ONLY SOLUTIONS

When you treat someone you never know how many 'anchors' there may be holding the patient's recovery back. And removing 99 per cent of the problems may still not produce a cure. You just have to keep looking for the last anchor. There always is one, you know. It just takes time, hard work and some luck to find it. Here are two examples of the puzzle-solving involved in treating patients, particularly those with CFS.

I was once worried about a patient, whom I'll call Tracy. I'd had only limited success in treating her, despite intensive efforts. An asthmatic, this young lady was very allergic and suffered from a viral illness. Her lifestyle was not the best: she smoked two packets of cigarettes per day, drank lots of alcohol and ate a diet heavy in red meats and fats. She was chronically tired.

After a week at a health farm, she improved considerably but, when she returned home could not stick to her new diet regimen and lifestyle. She resumed smoking, drinking lots of coffee, eating all sorts of junk food and boozing. Realising I was working uphill, as it were, I sent her for oxygen (ozone) therapy. After more than ten treatments she was poorer, but no better off.

In spite of the fact that she never experienced vaginal thrush and had few, if any, digestive symptoms, I decided to try some anti-fungal therapy usually reserved for people with candida. I also managed to get her to stop eating yeast-mould foods. Within a couple of weeks she was as good as new.

I also agonised over a CFS patient — we'll call her Mary — who was so sick she could not even lift a shopping bag with a bottle of milk in it. She had been unwell for several months after contracting a virus in Europe, and had relapsed into being very unwell in the previous three months. Feeling slightly feverish in spite of a normal temperature, she was anxious, depressed and at times did not even have the strength to chew her food. She had clear signs of Epstein Barr virus reactivation (with high VCA titres and a positive early antigen result).

In such cases the most useful treatment, in my experience, is a series of intravenous vitamin C (IVC) procedures. I have lost count of the people I have treated successfully with this method. Normally we start with a medium dose and then adjust both the frequency and dose according to the results. If the virus is already active success is measured by the improvement of the patient's condition. If the virus itself is inactive at the time (with test results showing negative early antigens and high viral capsid antigen titres), or if there is evidence of a poor original response to the viral attack (negative EBNA nuclear antigens) then success is shown by the patient experiencing a sudden onset or flare-up of flu-like symptoms, often including sore or swollen glands (lymphadenopathy).

Doses of vitamin C vary from 30 g to 120 g and the frequency from daily for five or more successive days to once in a while. Generally speaking viral CFS responds better to many consecutive treatments while chemical CFS may need high but infrequent procedures. We tried 60 g of vitamin C — it achieved nothing. So the dose was upped to 90 g. Zilch! A full 120 g helped for a couple of hours, after which Mary was worse than ever. I decided to try a massive dose of 180 g over a couple of hours. Mary responded as if she had been given an electric charge. She was well, had energy, most of her pains were gone but she was terribly restless and could hardly sleep at night. Within two days it all fell apart again and she was as bad as ever.

Mark Donohoe and I had a brainstorming session and discussed Mary's case. Why did Mary only respond to such a high dose and then only temporarily? We both knew that vitamin C, although always described as an antioxidant, is in fact an oxidator at small doses, an antioxidant at higher levels, but then an oxidator again beyond a certain point. Her response to the high level of vitamin C certainly seemed like the effects of oxygenation therapy!

There are many forms of oxygen therapy — oral, intravenous, etc. — and I remembered my previous failure with ozone therapy with Tracy, but nevertheless in desperation I decided to try it again.

Mary recovered almost miraculously after only one treatment! Yet her 'mental' symptoms did not. She was still somewhat anxious, depressed and moody. I gave her a large oral dose of a liquid zinc preparation. Within a couple of hours she was well emotionally as well as physically.

The next ozone procedure and a little more zinc made her as well as she could be! After about ten days, however, she began slowly to deteriorate again. I contacted Dr Ian Dettman in Melbourne, Victoria, who is the son of Glen Dettman, the Australian pioneer in orthomolecular and vitamin C research. From Ian I obtained information about his supply of hydrogen peroxide intravenous infusions. With the help of my Queensland associate, Dr Kevin Treacy, who administered the infusion, we started the therapy.

The next thing we knew was that Mary spent the weekend

dancing at a local disco until 3 a.m.!

This story just goes to show that you have to try every avenue; you have to pull up *all* the 'anchors' and you also have to remember that one method of treatment alone may not cause the desired response — it may be that it is one treatment on top of other procedures that finally works.

Doctors Talk to Doctors About CFS

Chronic Fatigue Syndrome

by Dr Mark Donohoe

CFS AND MODERN MEDICINE
Chronic Fatigue Syndrome (CFS) has proven as elusive and divisive an issue as exists in modern medical history. The roots and consequences of this division have tended to isolate those affected by the illness, to the extent that 'self-help' groups have become the major sources of information and the major impetus for continued research and investigation.

This is a significant departure from the perceived methods of assessment and progress within medicine, and has proven a blow to our professional pride. Traditionally, medicine is seen to be hierarchically driven from above. Information is passed from the pristine academic community, through the medical schools and medical journals, and eventually on to the overworked and under-trained primary practitioner. Here it remains, awaiting application of the knowledge when the appropriate patient fits the pattern. The patient has no part in this scheme, apart from being a passive, unquestioning consumer.

The truth is that, in an increasingly overcrowded medical community, and with an aware and well-educated public, the consumers drive the process, and are demanding to be included in the diagnostic process and the choice of appropriate therapy. Doctors are being asked to explain decisions and define choices, and the consumers are becoming 'clients' rather than 'patients'. Doctors are assuming their roles as teachers once again, working with clients as equals in the understanding and management of health problems. Consumers vote with their wallets, and those doctors unwilling to see the value and benefit of the new alliance with their clients are fossilising mentally, ignoring a golden opportunity for truly progressive change.

In fact, if there is a revolution within late twentieth century medicine, it is less the high tech, impersonal and costly wizardry, and more the discovery of our most under-utilised resource — the unwell person! In the rush towards 'science', we tended to ignore the patient as a resource. Patients, for their part, became the willing subjects of a medical community who promised to take away their pain, their diseases, and their responsibility for their own health. This was the 'golden age' of medicine, with unbounded promises and possibilities, and a world which hoped that all problems could be 'fixed' by the appropriate miracle. We did not have to care for ourselves — or so we hoped.

While not an overt hoax, it would be true to say that the expectations were unrealistic, yet little was done to place any 'scientific perspective' on this dream. Money flowed freely, and medicine became a new religion for many — belief and hope in no way matched by reality.

Literally trillions of dollars in the past 60 years have achieved much less than we would have hoped. Increased life expectancy has become the 'holy grail' of modern medicine, and the focus has been always on heroic efforts and medical miracles. In fact, the heroic face of medicine — the bone marrow transplants, heart transplants, trauma victims, liver transplants, and artificial organs — achieve virtually nothing in terms of improvement in quality of life or longevity of the general population, except to decrease it! This is the obscene public relations face of medicine, the front page tabloid entertainment. While it may allow us all to feel more secure that when all else fails, there will always be a medicine there to save us, like the knight in shining armour, in fact the reverse is true.

As Ivan Illich points out in *The Medical Nemesis*, medicine reaches its peak of effectiveness when it is able to distribute resources evenly and efficiently across the entire population. The inequity of these heroic measures concentrates massive resources on a few individuals, at a significant opportunity cost to the whole population. In this way, we risk the health of the whole by overvaluing the lives of the few!

Certainly, it is heartbreaking to see a 22-week, 400-gram premature baby die. On the grand scale, though, it is a travesty that more resources should be spent on the rescue of a single child than on the education and nutrition of ten thousand pregnant women. The outcome of the former, at best, is the salvage of a baby who will remain moderately or severely retarded lifelong, requiring special education, social security payments, and enormous family stresses for decades after the birth. The holy grail of 'life at any cost' has been achieved, and years have been added to this one life. What of the quality of life, though?

The best outcome of an education and dietary program for ten thousand women is less dramatic and less tangible, but is statistically demonstrable. A reduction in low birth-weight and premature babies in the order of tens to hundreds may reasonably be expected. With little drama, dozens of normal children take their place in families at no added cost to the community, and without anyone knowing which of those children would have been the damaged ones.

The problem is seen in stark relief. On one hand, the drama and emotional tug of a salvaged life — a story, a parable, and an expression of our collective hopes and dreams of victory over death. It mobilises funds, creates professional careers, and, in crude terms, is great copy. Politicians win votes by supporting the programs, and the medical community remains silent while the good press continues. There is no voice for 'good science' during the euphoria, no reminders of the 'limits to medicine'. On the other hand, the boredom of prevention galvanises nothing. Media have no pictures, no story line, no interest. Shoestring budgets administered by volunteers, employing barefoot doctors and nurses, are the norm, and politicians gain little by supporting invisible, though effective, measures.

Thus, the stage has been set for medicine to look towards dramatic, simple, single causes for all problems, and CFS sufferers are victims of this legacy. In a complex world, where most 'single agent disease' has found a cure of sorts, we are left with the messy, multi-factorial, degenerative problems. Attempts to ascribe a single agent to a complex illness, such as happened with HIV (Human Immunodeficiency Virus), are being shown to be progressively less tenable. HIV is a social problem, a community problem, a problem of attitudes, a drug problem, a prejudice problem and an infective problem. HIV is a part of the illness complex, but it was prematurity, prejudice and undue haste which led to both the disease (AIDS) and the virus sharing the same name. This effectively absolved us of our guilt, removed the need to look carefully at our lifestyles, and destroyed an opportunity for progress in health on many different levels. The virus and the disease became synonymous, and the answer became the technical search for a vaccine or curative medication. Depersonalised, the disease lost its meaning, and reduced sufferers to the position of total helplessness as they awaited the handing down of the next ray of scientific hope. For once, this was not forthcoming, and people began to die of hopelessness as much as of the virus.

Yet, as Dr Al Levin, a San Francisco immunologist and primary AIDS practitioner for a large HIV-positive community, said as far back as 1988, 'HIV is an eminently manageable condition — all that is required is a few simple medications and a total change of attitudes and lifestyle!'

Giving meaning to the illnesses which people suffer has been part of the human heritage since the dawn of history, and in every culture. From cave dwellers through all the great civilisations, and from Hippocrates to the pre-war herbalist or medical practitioner, there lived a dynamic wisdom in the understanding and management of disease and pain. There was little of scientific merit to be done, so we listened, laughed, cried and shared in the process. The healer was revered, not because of science, but because he or she gave meaning to the illness and the person, and placed them in the context of their own community. The person became whole again, whether or not they recovered from the illness. This belonging and integration is critical to recovery and to maintaining health. We must never forget our roots — linguistic or historical. 'Health' is derived from 'whole', and 'doctor' is the Latin term for 'teacher'.

Too often today we confuse 'healthy' with 'not sick'. We see ourselves in the medical profession as the technical administrators of a scientific discipline, and believe that symptomatic management and appropriate therapy will create health. We may do the opposite. The removal of symptoms may leave the person in limbo, not sick in any life threatening way (and we *do* still measure our success in terms of life duration), but not healthy.

Further, these people are left isolated by their own community and eventually their own family, because they have no name, no validation, and no context for their ill health. They become misfits, eschewed by the medical community which turns the blame back on the unwell person ('It's all in your mind', 'Well, you did bring it on yourself', or 'You're just depressed'), and lost to their family and community who cannot understand this state, who can find no comfortable place for them, and who can develop no relationship or role with them. They become the modern 'untouchables', more because of our fear of the unknown than because of the severity of the disability.

It has been said that modern medicine is the victory of cleverness over wisdom. We hoped that an impersonal, objective, and statistical science would remove the need for human contact and understanding. The five-minute consultation and the prescription pad are the symbols and the icons of this faith. In a belated Newtonian carry-over, we hoped that humans were like clocks, albeit more complex. We believed in linear and predictable systems, and became confused about statistics. We began to approach everyone in the same way, and devalued communication, caring, empathy and 'the common touch'. We became technocrats, and threw away our heritage, our art.

I will confess now my passionate love for science and the scientific method, possibly the greatest creation of the human mind in all history. I am constantly excited by its achievements and its creations. I believe in science, and it must form the basis of our health care. To not use and apply good science is a tragedy that we cannot afford. The critical term, though, is 'good science'. This implies an open mind, observation, intellectual freedom, hypothesis, testing, and application. Good science is no more a double-blind trial than a good car is a good engine. Progress occurs with the meeting of facts and the well prepared and open mind. If we do not look, we will never see, and it bothers me when 'science' opposes the right of people to hold certain concepts and opinions, especially when it is the academics who oppose the ideas of field workers. The risk is that specialisation in medicine may break down our ability to appreciate whole people, for while we are good at pulling things apart and analysing, we are not proficient at the re-assembly of these facts to a meaningful whole. The re-assembly is the synthesis, the art of medicine. The analysis is the science. Careful balancing of the two, in ways appropriate to the individual, is the wisdom of our profession, and it is time we relearned valuable old skills.

It is now time to reclaim the art, the humanity of our profession, and to marry it to the science. The trillions of dollars have extended quality and quantity of life only marginally, despite the apparent differences in raw figures. Agricultural changes, sanitation, sewerage, fresh clean water, building codes and safe birthing practices have done more to extend quality and quantity of life than *any* of our modern miracles, including antibiotics.

Survival at birth is the major statistical extender of life statistics. A single child who would have died, but who lives to 70 because of improved birth practices is statistically much more important than the 58 year old overweight smoker whose life is extended two years with triple bypass surgery. And so it should be. But the premature child who lives, brain damaged, to 70 in an institution also improves the statistics in the short term, equally with the normal child.

As a 20 year old in 1976, my expected further life duration of 50-odd years (taking me to 70 or so) was only an improvement of two years in a 20 year old in 1926 (when the effects of two world wars are taken into account). Yet in my final 10 to 12 years, I could now be expected to be affected by degenerative disease of some type — cardiovascular, arthritic or cancer. As a 20 year old back in 1926, I could expect 6 to 8 years of this type of illness. I am now more likely to be medicated, operated upon, investigated and suffer side effects of medical treatment than in the 1920s.

In short, I will probably live longer, but will likely be in worse health for longer, requiring more costly medications. Is this worth the trillions spent? Would this money have been better spent on the basics of agriculture, food distribution, sanitation and the like in Third World countries, and improved nutrition in all countries? History will be the judge, but my feeling is that we have lost a golden opportunity, possibly forever.

It is within this context, and with this personal perspective that I wish to preface the information that will follow in this chapter. I shall be dealing with this condition in a somewhat technical manner, and I believe it is vital not to perpetuate the myth that CFS is a purely technical illness. It is an illness of the cell membranes, the nerves and lymphocytes, the brain and bowel, the person, their family, their community, our society, our culture, and even our planet. On every level, it is possible to see the connections with all the other levels, and these connections become more obvious and complex the more one deals with the disease. So, while technical aspects and hypotheses are vitally important, they are NOT the disease itself.

My background in this field is one of six years of general practice with a major interest in listening to people! My practice was in an area of New South Wales already grossly overstocked with medical practitioners, and in a location with no more than a few hundred local inhabitants. My daughter, Misha, was six months old, and I knew little enough about business to take out a sizeable loan, outfit a building, and spend hours listening to people.

I kept listening and documenting, and a pattern emerged. People were coming from everywhere with the symptoms of weakness, fatigue, myalgia, allergies and numerous other symptoms which later were grouped together as CFS. My practice grew in five years to nearly 2000 families, coming from throughout New South Wales and even interstate, and my waiting list extended to many months. And this was in spite of the fact that I could do little or nothing for the illness.

In 1985 I first read the articles in *Annals of Internal Medicine* by Jones et al, and by Straus et al, on 'Chronic or Persistent Epstein-Barr Infection'. Suddenly, I realised that I was not alone, and jumped on the diagnosis as a quick answer for a complex problem. I performed the antibody studies and many of my clients did, indeed, fit the criteria. But many did not!

It was around this time that I first met William Vayda. William Vayda is unique, and has probably the most voracious appetite for information and understanding of anyone I have known. His ability to absorb and link information from various sources over periods of years is of continuing amazement to me, and his skill in presenting the information in an entertaining and simplified way in his articles and lectures gives his ideas relevance and reach.

I have been working with William Vayda over the past five years on and off, and his practice comprises the broadest range of clinical conditions one could ever hope to see. People come from around Australia and from overseas, having been through the whole medical machine without satisfaction. I act as a consultant on medical aspects of the illnesses I see there, and while differences of opinion are not uncommon (with my Irish background and his Hungarian background, this is not surprising!), the intellectual stimulation of working with Vayda and in his clinic has helped mould many of the ideas and concepts outlined here. I have learned not to judge by appearances, for this rough diamond is the intellectual superior of any university lecturer or professor I have ever known in terms of breadth of knowledge, synthesis of new ideas, safe application of the ideas, and ability to achieve results where so many others have failed.

In mid 1989 I joined up with Drs Dobie, Fluhrer and Marshall to design and create an allergy unit, where the principles of withdrawal and challenge could be applied for foods, chemical solvents, and food chemicals in a controlled and modified environment setting. This was opened in October 1989 at the Manly Waters Hospital in New South Wales, and was christened the Special Environment Allergy Clinic (SEAC, pronounced *'seek'*). Drs Dobie, Fluhrer and I man the Environmental Medicine Centre Outpatients Department (OPD), and have done so since September 1990 in response to the high demand for places on the ward, and an increasing number of doctors requiring a point for referral of clients who they believe may be environmentally affected. The SEAC is currently expanding to simply keep up with demand.

In these seven years, I have seen over 1000 CFS sufferers according to the strict diagnostic criteria of the time, and hundreds more who seem to have CFS, but lack one or more of the essential diagnostic criteria. My focus and interest has been more on those with past chemical exposure or those with chemical hypersensitivity syndrome (CHS) and allergy, and this may make the CFS clients I see different from other groups. I include this background and disclaimer to draw attention to the direction from which I approach this disease, and to highlight any differences between the information I have accumulated over time, and the general medical and scientific experience with the illness. The presented information is a synthesis of my own experience and a broad literature base, current at early 1991.

Further, I have decided not to include a bibliography or reading list with this chapter, which is intended more as an introduction and primer for those who have a medical or technical interest in CFS and related conditions. There are numerous articles and books suitable for various levels of technical proficiency, and an appropriate reading list can be provided for a few dollars for anyone interested, simply by contacting The Complementary Medicine Centre, 41 Boundary St, Rushcutters Bay, NSW 2011, Australia, or The Environmental Medicine Centre, Manly Waters Private Hospital, 17 Cove Ave, Manly, NSW 2095, Australia. Continued presentation of findings from both Centres will occur at regular intervals for practitioners with a continuing interest.

TYPICAL SYMPTOMATOLOGY OF CFS
Hallmarks of the Condition and Diagnosis

There is only one universal symptom of CFS — fatigue! Various other symptoms are present in individuals at various probabilities, commonly around 70 per cent to 90 per cent prevalence. A summary of these is listed below, taken from the data presented in the June 1990 *Journal of Clinical Microbiology*.

Clinical symptomatology of patients with CFS expressed as percentage of symptoms manifested

Symptom	% of patients
Fatigue	100
Low-grade fever	85
Sore throat	76
Adenopathy	40
Painful lymph nodes	30
Unexplained general muscle weakness	90
Myalgias	90
Prolonged fatigue (more than 24 hours after exercise)	80
Headaches	76
Arthralgias	90
Photophobia (light sensitivity)	76
Inability to concentrate	90
Forgetfulness	90
Irritability	85

Confusion	90
Mood swings	90
Emotional lability	90
Depression	80
Difficulty sleeping	76
Ability to date onset of illness	100
Gastrointestinal complaints	30
Shortness of breath	33
Allergies	70
Hot flushes	30
Vertigo	40
Nausea	33
Palpitations	30
Chest pain	33
Night sweats	25
Weight loss	80
Weight gain	15
Rash	15

CFS remains in 1991 a diagnosis of exclusion, and primary practitioners are under increasing pressure to arrive at a diagnosis with minimum expenditure.

There is a diagnostic 'break-even point' in CFS, but it varies according to the perceptions of the practitioner and the history and demographics of the client. Many practitioners will diagnose CFS on the history of persistent weakness and fatigue, but this ignores other possibilities such as hypothyroidism, anaemia, metabolic abnormalities, other endocrine conditions, and major primary psychiatric disorders such as unipolar or bipolar affective depressive disorders.

Others, such as immunologists and specialist referral practices (such as my own), are required to do more. Possible other serious illness must be excluded, and the pattern of immunological, neuropsychological, and other tests must point positively to a likely or plausible causative agent. I have seen people referred with 'CFS for investigation' with a broad range of other pathology, including Cushings Syndrome, ulcerative colitis, adrenal tumors, mitral valve disease, severe cardiovascular disease, brucellosis, simple anaemia, lymphoma and other malignancies, and inappropriate or excessive medication.

RULE 1: *Any intercurrent medical condition should be identified and treated prior to management of CFS.*

If in doubt, refer the client to an immunologist or specialist CFS clinic, who can apply more extensive investigations without fear of government intervention.

Although CDC have a good working case definition, my preference is for the definition of the Prince Henry/Prince of Wales group in Sydney. In substance, the definitions are the same, but the criteria are easier to apply and more relevant, and psychiatric dysfunction (such as depression) is not an exclusion criterion.

This is an important question on a practical and philosophical level. Which diagnosis takes precedence, CFS or depression?

Most, if not all, people with chronic illness show intermittent or constant depressive tendencies. This is a natural consequence of chronic illness on both a physiological and psychological level, and is understandable. A positive diagnosis of, say, heart disease provides a context for the depression, and validates (or normalises) the psychological state. Clients are not referred to psychiatrists and are not medicated for the depression. The focus is on the underlying illness, as it should be. Resources are mobilised, and care is forthcoming from the community. This tends to alleviate the isolation and pain, and the depression subsides further. This is true even in cases of inevitably fatal illness, such as terminal cancer.

On the other hand, a person with CFS does not yet have a positive diagnosis at the time they are referred for psychiatric assessment. They are weak and depressed, and are said to have 'no physical basis for their complaints'. In such a context, the psychological state becomes the focus of investigation, and it is not unusual to find symptoms which support the diagnosis of depression. Two points are missed in this approach, however. The very pathogenesis of the disease proposed in the immunological and neurological models predicts positively that depression is a symptom of the underlying disorder. Interferon, interleukins and inflammatory mediators cause depression when given to healthy volunteers, and are a major side effect in, say, the use of interferon in hairy cell leukaemia and chronic hepatitis. The toxic neurological effects of solvents include depression and memory loss, and many medications are capable of inducing clinically significant depression.

In my opinion, the diagnosis of CFS should be part of the differential diagnosis in depression, with a known or proposed physical cause for depression taking precedence over the proposed mysterious appearance of the psychological state. Depression, as a psychiatric diagnosis, cannot be disproved, and becomes the opinion of the practitioner assessing the person. Evidence cannot be brought from objective testing which is capable of falsifying the assertion of depression as a diagnosis. In this sense, psychiatry is generally poor science, in that it is unable to fulfil the major requirement of good science — that of being able to define an objective standard to demonstrate the fallacy of a proposal or assertion.

Practitioners working with CFS do not have this luxury of assertion creating reality. We are eternally pushed to define objective tests which, depending on the result, tend to confirm or deny the likelihood of the diagnosis. In such a setting, precedence and preference should be given to the position with best evidence, positive or negative. Depression, therefore, should not be diagnosed unless an attempt has been made to exclude CFS as a more plausible diagnosis.

RULE 2: *Except in the case of depressive affective disorders (psychotic depression) the diagnosis of CFS is to be preferred to depression as a primary diagnosis.*

DIAGNOSIS — THE PRINCIPLES AND METHODS
A person presenting with fatigue who fits the following general case definition is likely to have CFS, and deserves further workup.

MAJOR CRITERIA
- Chronic persisting or relapsing fatigue, generalised in nature, exacerbated by minor exercise, present for more than six months, and causing significant disruption of usual daily activities.
- Neuropsychiatric dysfunction including significant impairment of concentration, and short-term memory impairment.
- Abnormal cell mediated immunity (CMI) evidenced by alteration of Natural Killer (NK) cell, T8 or T4 lymphocyte subset numbers or function, and/or cutaneous anergy or hypoergy on Multitest CMI.

SUPPORTIVE FINDINGS
Symptoms lasting more than six months, consistently or intermittently, of three or more of the following — myalgia, arthralgia, headaches, sleep disturbance, paraesthesiae, tinnitus, or depression.
Signs (present on two or more occasions during initial illness): lymphadenopathy, lymphodynia, pharyngitis, localised muscle tenderness (one or more).

Thus, history taking is the primary tool of diagnosis in CFS, and is the most cost-effective means of diagnosis available. The only tool required is an open mind!

However, the history should include information beyond the usual medical history, and may take upwards of 30 minutes to be done properly. It should include a complete environmental survey, including allergy, sensitivities, occupational survey, home survey, assessment of accidental or occupational toxic exposure to any agents, and a lifestyle survey including weight, height, body-mass index (BMI), and assessment of fitness and exercise.

From this point, how is the average practitioner to exclude other possible causes, and provide positive evidence for the diagnosis?

The following table gives a brief summary of the pathology and other testing which has generally proven to be useful in the working through of this illness, with notes about any which are less usual or difficult to perform:

Initial Investigation (exclude other common causes of symptoms)

Test	Notes
FBC (full blood count)	Good basic screen
TFTs & TSH	Exclude overt hypothyroidism
ANA	Autoimmune assessment
LFTs, biochem	Exclude specific endorgan disease
White cell diff	Identify leukocytosis, leukopenia
Paul-Bunnell	Exclude initial acute EBV
IgE	Exclude allergy
RAST	MX-1, FX-5, GX-2, HX-2 basic allergy screen
B-12 & RC Folate	Exclude nutritional deficiency

Ferritin, Fe Stud.	Exclude iron deficiency
CXR	Exclude TB, sarcoidosis, infection
Skin Allergy Tests	Specific antigenic reactions, IgE based
Multitest CMI	Assess CMI (see below)
Cardiologist	Cardiological assessment (especially mitral valve disease)

This will, in the majority of cases, exclude most significant other causes of the symptoms of CFS, but not all. A more complete survey may then be undertaken to attempt to positively identify possible causative agents, including:

Test	Notes
EBV studies	VCA-IgG, AEA, EBNA, and IgM - ?CEBV
CMV	IgG & IgM
Toxoplasmosis	IgG & IgM
Ross River Virus	IgG & IgM
Hepatitis serology	Hep A & B (?Hep C in transfusions)
Brucellosis	Other relevant Zoonoses as well

If doubt persists about the existence of an immune deficiency state, it is worth referring the client for immunological studies, including studies of lymphocyte subset numbers, functional tests of immune activity, and exclusion of more exotic illnesses.

Should all of these prove unhelpful in determining the cause of the immune-deficiency or fatigue syndrome, assessment of blood or tissue levels of potentially immunotoxic agents should be considered. This is often best done in a specialist clinic, after a full occupational workup, and with specialised collection methods.

Possible agents which can cause health problems which mimic CFS include:

- *Heavy metals (Hg, Pb, As, Cd, Al)* through enzyme blockade
- *Organochlorine pesticides (HCB, dieldrin, DDT analogues, etc.)* through direct and indirect long term immunotoxicity
- *PCBs through occupational exposure* (electricians, merchant ship seamen)

- *Organophosphorous pesticides (dichlorvos, etc.)* through multiple esterase inhibition in nerve, muscle, intracellular enzyme systems
- *Aliphatic solvents (hexane, etc.) and aromatic solvents (toluene, etc.)* in disturbance of renal or hepatic function, and direct neuro- and immuno-toxicity
- *Halogenated solvents (Carbon tetrachloride, chloroform, 1,1,1-TCE)* via similar (though more potent) pathways of other solvents above
- *Chlorinated phenols (pentachlorophenol)* through enzyme blockade
- *Dioxins and dibenzo furans* through intracellular hormonal and DNA disrupting pathways
- *Quaternary ammonia products and cationic surfactants* through disruption of cell membranes.

Many of these products are capable of inducing free radical production in their breakdown and detoxication, and lipid peroxidation at this point produces malonaldehyde, a potent carcinogen. It is at this point that antioxidant therapy may be of greatest use.

While not all can be tested, a clear exposure history along with typical symptoms will in many cases suffice, and detoxication can be commenced with appropriate agents.

At this stage, most reversible causes of the condition will have been excluded, and the diagnosis of CFS will be fairly well established. However, it is impossible to leave the subject of diagnosis without at least a passing mention of *Candida albicans*, and its part in the generation of this illness.

In truth, 'candidiasis' has become the uncritical catch-cry of many sufferers and consumers alike, and has the difficulty of being essentially an almost impossible to test hypothesis. To this end, it is useful only in as much as it may lead to a dose of nystatin, and many people do improve on this regimen. This is NOT science, but a seat-of-the-pants method of improving the health of some people who otherwise remain unwell.

It seems, from my experience, that the syndrome is real, but has been grossly overdiagnosed and treated without critical thought. While Dr Vayda has dealt with this matter extensively, a simple observation is in order here. The people who have most relief of symptoms from the use of nystatin and dietary manipulation seem to be those who suffer T-cell immune deficiency and allergy to moulds simultaneously. These people come up positive to various moulds on RAST testing and skin sensitivity testing, and commonly undergo an initial adverse reaction on commencing nystatin (the so-called die-off, or herxheimer reaction).

Thus, it is less a matter of the virulence of the candida organism (which is ubiquitous) than it is a matter of decreased host defences, and host hypersensitivity to the cytoplasmic or cell wall components. These two states, simultaneously, diminish the cell mediated control of the organism in its invasive (filamentous) state, and allow for chronic inflammatory allergic reactions on the gut wall, leading to many of the symptoms attributed to food allergy. The symptoms disappear over time with avoidance of yeast antigens in the diet, anti-fungal therapy, or allergy immunotherapy.

I have no doubt that for this smaller subset of CFS sufferers, antifungal therapy is of immense importance in the regaining of normal gastrointestinal function, and decrease in allergenic loads, and the method of treatment is safe and has few side effects.

One further area of controversy is the area of hormonal dysregulation in this illness. Many sufferers appear clearly hypothyroid, with the full gamut of myxadematous symptoms, yet TSH and TFTs are normal. Good medical practice states that these people should not be treated with thyroid supplementation (thyroxine).

The problem is that many of these people, when treated empirically with thyroxine, do improve in symptoms in both the short and long term, but not until very high doses are reached in some cases. Others improve at low doses of 50 μg or below. This is an area certainly worthy of further study, as there is a model with another common hormonal disorder, diabetes. In many of these people, the circulating hormone is at normal or even high levels, but the cells are unable to respond to the hormone due to damaged hormonal receptors. The same may be occurring in this so called 'peripheral hypothyroidism', and monoclonal markers for peripheral Thyroxine and T3 receptors would be of enormous benefit.

In the meantime, any approach with supplemental thyroxine in these circumstances is experimental, and must never be tried without full consent and with the person under constant supervision. Assessment of dosage is done on clinical grounds, and the hormonal assays are not a reliable indicator of hormonal adequacy.

APPLICATION AND INTERPRETATION OF TESTS
Multitest CMI

Multitest CMI testing shows a definite, strongly negative correlation with the presence of symptoms of CFS (i.e. more severe and frequent symptoms are associated with a lower total score), and is a cost-effective screening method for depressed cell mediated immune function.

The Multitest CMI is a standard item able to be ordered through any pharmacy, though it should be applied and read by those experienced and trained in its use. It has been part of the immunological workup of every client in our SEAC since its opening in late 1989, and should become as much a part of every medical practitioner's diagnostic process as the ECG or pathology testing.

The Multitest itself is a means of applying seven antigens and a glycerine control intradermally, via the use of pre-loaded wells of antigen on a small plastic carrier. The wells are uncovered prior to application, the skin of the forearm near the elbow crease is prepared with an alcohol swab and allowed to dry thoroughly, and the Multitest is then applied firmly to this skin with the 'T' end of the device 5 cm below the elbow crease. After 5 to 10 seconds of firm application, the Multitest is discarded (it MUST NOT BE RE-USED on another subject, and should not be re-applied to the same subject, even if you cannot see fluid on the arm where it has been applied). The area is kept open during the subsequent 10 minutes to allow evaporation of the antigens, and should not be covered by a sleeve or wiped in this time, to prevent possible mixing and contamination of antigens. A skin marker is applied to the position of the 'T' section to allow for later antigen identification and scoring. The whole process sounds dauntingly difficult, but is in fact no more than a two-minute procedure, and is an astonishingly simple test for the information it gives.

The reading of the Multitest is done at exactly 48 hours in order to standardise results. While it may be of interest to note which antigens caused immediate (Type-I, allergic) reactivity, and which ones led to erythema, the only measurement required is the measurement of the *number* and *size* of indurated (thickened, raised and reddish) responses. Each indurated mark is measured in two axes, and the average of these two measurements is the size (in millimetres) for that antigen. Each is recorded on a standard score sheet, and the final score is recorded as 'XX/ Y', where XX is the total of all the sizes, and Y is the number of antigens which recorded a positive result.

So, what information does it give? The Multitest is an *in vivo* test of cell mediated (largely T-cell) immune function. It measures the ability of T-lymphocytes to respond to particular antigenic stimulation, lymphocyte transformation, and lymphocyte migration. In basic terms, it is largely the cell mediated branch of the immune system which is responsible for long-term memory and management of viruses, pathogenic fungi, and many malignancies.

It is a test of so-called 'Type-IV' hypersensitivity, and tends to increase with age in a population up to age 20 or so. Men have generally higher results than women by approximately one antigen and 5 mm.

As far as interpretation of results goes, an amount of 05/1 is added to the female scores (to allow for sex differences), and interpretation is done on this final figure. 'Anergy' is defined as a 'score' of 05/2 or less (i.e. 5 mm total size of indurations, 2 antigens positive). 'Hyopergy', or relative anergy, is defined as above 05/2 but less than or equal to 10/3. These values are for adults, though there are many journal articles available from the manufacturer giving average scores (and spread) for various age groups and sex.

Epstein-Barr Virus (EBV)
While complex, the following is a simple summary of the likely causes of various combinations of EBV antibody studies. It is probably true that EBV is not the causative agent in the majority of CFS sufferers, but assessment of the antibody status is a valuable guide to native immune function.

The antibodies in question are the viral capsid antigen IgG (VCA-IgG), anti early antigen (AEA), nuclear antigen (EBNA) and specific IgM. The VCA is given as a titration value, while the AEA is assessed at a titre of 1:80 and measured positive or negative. The EBNA is measured similarly at a 1:10 dilution. These are done with the FDA approved du Pont test kit.

The normal state for anyone who has never been exposed to the EB virus is that all antigens are negative, and the person is commonly well. Over 99 per cent of Western world inhabitants have been exposed to the EB virus by age 25 to 30, and as an 'immortal' herpes virus, it has the capacity for long life and immune reactivation.

The following brief guide leaves out many details, but is used for simplicity:

VCA IgG	EBNA	AEA	IgM	Interpretation
160-640	+	–	–	Normal post-exposure state
variable	–	–	+	Acute early EBV
>640	–	+	+	Acute EBV (2-4 weeks)
>640	+	–	–	Recovery from acute EBV (3 months)
>2560	+	+	±	Likely chronic or recurrent EBV
>2560	–	+	±	CEBV with poor initial immune response
<160	–	+	+	Relapse of EBV in immune deficiency states

PROPOSED CAUSES

Controversies abound in medical circles when the talk turns to CFS, but in no area is the discussion more lively than that of the cause of the illness.

There is no single known cause for the disease, and no one candidate seems more likely than others to assume dominance in the foreseeable future. Most of the medical establishment's money is on one of the many common viruses, including EBV, human herpes virus 6 (HHV-6), coxsaccie B virus, cytomegalovirus, or even a relative of the T-lymphotrophic viruses (the group to which Robert Gallo mistakenly attributed the AIDS virus). CFS has even been termed 'AIDS-free AIDS' because of initial apparent similarities between it and the early stages of HIV.

Data from our Special Environment Allergy Clinic at Manly tend to support the concept that a persistent viral infection is a common (though not universal) phenomenon in this disease. Our findings concur with those of a paper in the *Journal of Clinical Microbiology* in June 1990, showing raised Natural Killer (NK) cell (CD-56) numbers, with decreased NK activity and cytotoxicity. Suppressor (CD-8) lymphocytes are generally raised in numbers, with normal or low helper (CD-4) lymphocytes, all as measured in peripheral blood.

What follows is a simple list of proposed aetiological agents, or contributing factors in CFS. All are covered in the text of the rest of Dr Vayda's book, and no in-depth discussion will be undertaken here:

Cellular Damage
- Free radicals and lipid peroxidation
- Membrane damage
- Enzyme damage or deficiency
- Mitochondrial and oxidative damage
- Decreased expression of DNA (hypomethylation)

Immunological Disorder
- Derangement of specific T-cell function
- Interleukin and general leukotreine abnormalities
- Genetically based immunodeficiency state

Chronic Opportunistic Infections
- Viral
    EBV
    CMV
    Coxsaccie B virus
    Ross River Virus
    Human Herpes VI
    HTLV
    Hep A, B, C
    HIV and 'AIDS-free AIDS'

- Bacterial
    - Abscesses (dental, bone, etc.)
    - Persistent streptococcal and staph infections
    - Chronic sinusitis (see below)
- Zoonoses and parasites
    - Toxoplasmosis and *Toxocara canis*
    - Brucellosis
- Pathogenic fungi
    - *Candida albicans*
    - Trichophyton

Allergy and Intolerance
- IgE mediated inhalant and food
- Mould Allergy and Chemical Hypersensitivity Syndrome
- Non-IgE mediated food and chemical sensitivities

Psychological Stress

Chemical toxicity
- Acute chemical toxicity (accidental)
- Chronic chemical toxicity and immunotoxicity
- Occupational exposure

Chemical Hypersensitivity Syndrome (CHS)
- Relationship with mould allergy

Nutritional Deficiency
- Micronutrients
    - Selenium (especially in Australia and NZ)
    - Zinc
    - Fatty acids omega-3, omega-6, GLA
- Protein-calorie deficiency
    - Especially after elimination diets
- Conversion of amino acids
    - Brain peptides production enzyme blockade
    - Detox peptides (GSH)
    - Gut oligopeptides (VIP, CCK)

Hormonal Dysregulation
- Damage to glands
- Damage to pituitary

- Damage to hypothalamus and diencephalon
- Damage to cellular receptors
   Thyroid hormone
- Idiotypes and anti-idiotype antibodies

Miscellaneous
- Chronic sinusitis (often 'silent')
- Mercury amalgam fillings
- Electromagnetic fields and ELF radiation

THERAPEUTIC INTERVENTION
Any of the principles of specific intervention are covered in the body of Dr Vayda's book. While there is no specific therapy which has proven universally successful in CFS, the following summary delineates certain approaches which have proven beneficial in some cirumstances.

Some of these approaches are used within our clinics, but the description of the application of these interventions in modification of the illness is beyond the scope of this chapter.

General Principles
1. Avoidance of all identified noxious and allergenic agents should be attempted, where possible. Known initiating factors should be minimised, and the principles of adequate rest, sleep, nutrition and more rest should be observed.
2. A brief elimination diet is certainly worth a trial under a dietitian's care, as is a program for attainment of ideal weight with good nutrition.
3. The person should be given reassurance that they are not alone, and that they will not be isolated, nor will they die or remain sick forever. The simple provision of a true diagnosis is often effective in helping the person come to grips with his or her symptoms, and begin to re-establish a normal life, with provisions for the illness.
4. Employers or school and the family should be included in the planning of a lifestyle compatible with recovery. The client may be unable to work for a considerable period, and community help and social security should be arranged at this time.

Protection
- Should be undertaken prior to and during any significant detox or immune modulation to minimise adverse reactions
- Oral ascorbate 1 to 4 g twice daily
- Sodium selenite 80–250 μg/day on empty stomach
- L-Cysteine or Methionine 500 mg — 2 twice daily between meals
- Vitamin E 500–750 IU daily
- Antioxidant combination formula (e.g. Proxidin 3 daily)
- Rest and time off work if possible for six weeks

Detoxification (if chemical toxicity is contributing to total load)
Depending on the xenobiotics which may require detoxification, various agents and modalities are used. Many of these can only be carried out under supervision in hospital, while others are simpler and can be done even at home. Generally, we admit clients to the SEAC should they need to undergo formal detoxification.

Note: Any person undertaking a detox program of this sort should do so ONLY under strict medical supervision, and following tests of kidney function and heart function by a medical practitioner.

- Massage — progressing from light to deep over three weeks — daily 30 minutes
- Sauna — dry heat, 60°C — progressing from 5 to 30 minutes 2–3 times daily
- Exercise — progressive aerobic exercise 15 to 90 minutes daily
- Supervised fat reduction under dietitian — 5 per cent reduction over 3 weeks
- IV ascorbate — 30 to 90 g — 1–3 times weekly over three weeks
- EDTA (heavy metals), N-acetyl cysteine (hepatotoxins) and/or other agents may be used depending on the specific needs.
- Supplements — oral vitamin C, vitamin E, selenium, cysteine, essential fatty acids, reverse osmosis water, vitamin B3, B1, B6, zinc and antioxidants

Immune Modulation
- Gamma globulin IV ('intragram') — 100 mls–500 mls — monthly x 3

- Gamma globulin IM — 5 mls–10 mls — weekly x 8
- Intravenous ascorbate — 30 g–150 g — 2 or 3 times, week 1
  Repeat same dose x 1–2 in weeks 2 and 3
- Budodouze forte IM (B1, B6, B12) — one weekly

Educate
A unifying educational program is essential to a good long-term prognosis in CFS. Initiating and contributing agents should be identified and modified, and the practitioner is in the position to co-ordinate the disparate information and to set realistic goals with the client.

Minimising the total load is a critical aspect of this approach, so as many of the stressors as possible should be identified, and decisions made with regard to the effort required in changing these factors.

Allergy management is instituted with allergen avoidance and specific imunotherapy if required. Information regarding minimising/avoiding xenobiotic chemicals at work and at home should be given, and consideration may need to be given to changing jobs.

CONCLUSION

At the end of the day, treatment may involve all or none of the above factors, for this is a person who is unwell, working in partnership with a supportive practitioner. It is not a disease requiring an academic, objective treatment.

Our ability to come to grips with this multifactorial and often frustrating illness will prove a watershed in medicine, a turning from the simple, didactic, linear models of decades past, to a new stable position of a mature ability to deal with complex, chaotic problems with co-operation and compassion.

The tools above are nothing more or less than that — tools. We are in a people business, and as healers and teachers, we owe our livelihood and art to those frustratingly wonderful people we used to call 'patients'.

Psychoneuroimmunology
by Dr Michael Glasby

Research is essentially a conversation with nature and like any good conversation, good research hinges on good questions.

Charles Sherrington

Research done last century showed that if you removed the right testicle a part of the left brain shrank. As interesting was evidence for the reverse effect, that is, if that part of the brain was operated on the testicle shrivelled. This may not seem to be relevant to a discussion on CFS, but, as I will show, it helps us to understand that the human body is not as simple as we might like to think. We learn in medical school that the immune system is an autonomous defence and protection mechanism, with relatively well understood mechanisms for activity and regulation. Modern research indicates that this 'simple' picture is no longer applicable, that the interconnectedness of the immune system with the neural and endocrine systems impels us to formulate new models which start to diverge from the mechanistic/reductionistic models still held widely today.

The idea that states of mind affect health was observed by Galen in the second century BC, in his finding that depressed women were more prone to breast cancer than their cheerful counterparts. The role of personality and adaptation to life was considered central to health up to the time of Descartes in the seventeenth century. The development of the current mind–body dualism was strengthened by the subsequent findings that external agents such as bacteria and viruses are direct causes of disease. Although these have been important steps brought about by the scientific approach they have driven the wedge in an old understanding based on observation, that the mind has profound effects on the body.

Now that we have an ability to research constitutional and behavioural factors in disease we can compare them with known disease-causing agents. One of the most revolutionary has been that published by H. J. Eysenck[1], in a study looking at people over a period of time — one of the most respected research techniques — which showed that not only were the researchers able to predict which personality types were likely to get cancer and heart disease but that they were stronger predictors than smoking, at least for lung cancer. More importantly, they had a control group that had experienced a period of counselling, and this was a significant prevention of both of these major illnesses.

Results of this nature have been available for many years. As long ago as 1960 Dr D. Kissen in Glasgow was able to differentiate men with lung cancer from those with other lung diseases by statistically significant psychological factors, such as an inability to express emotions. These older studies were criticised as being invalid for various reasons. These reasons have been overcome by more recent work, clearly showing the intricate relationship between mind and body.

Charmaine was a very able nurse with a long list of problems. Using the approach set out in Dr Vayda's book we were able together to bring her to a state of relative well-being over a period of three months.

She came to see me on short notice one day complaining of feeling terrible, but there were no obvious factors that she could recognise. After some discussion it became clear to me that her problem emanated from a deterioration in her relationship with a nephew. She had been very close to him because of some problems they both shared. Her brother was having some difficulties not only financially, but mostly with the son she was close to. Her brother was bringing these problems to the family, and Charmaine's previously very good relationship with her nephew was affected because he thought she was taking the side of his father. As we talked about how she felt about this division she understood the effect that this stressor had on her and we developed techniques to help her remain uninvolved in the negative aspects of her brother's problem, and thus restore the relationship with her nephew.

This is not an isolated incident. Those of us working in the area of counselling deal with such situations on a daily basis. Whether it's with family, friends, work or neighbours, negative ways of dealing with relationship stresses are a common cause of feeling bad. I say this with a degree of caution as causation within medicine is a 'protected' word, which requires clear statistical proof. As clearly as we see people feel better when we get them to respond in a different way to stressors, then just as clearly we can say that stress is causal to deterioration in many conditions.

THE CURRENT VIEW OF THE IMMUNE SYSTEM

Since Descartes, science has worked with the idea that to understand the 'big picture', one has to examine the components of the system in ever-increasing detail — the so-called Cartesian notion of reductionism. Coupled with this is a mechanistic view that cause-and-effect rules apply to body systems. This implies to some extent that the brain controls thinking and that there are clear mechanisms of control within body systems, consisting of specialised anatomically defined organ(s).

Immunologist R. Booth[2] develops the rationale that the immune system as a system at war with invaders (consisting of viruses, bacteria, etc.) is no longer a tenable model. He questions the ability of the medical fraternity to work with models; rather they prefer to follow, or have only been shown, philosophical strategies more related to those associated with dogma. Current views hold that disease is an unnatural state, caused by infectious agents which must be fought by the immune system, which operates as a defence mechanism, autonomous and essentially self regulating, discriminating between the body and foreign materials in a continuous battle to maintain health, and that the extremes of life are associated with an inability of the immune system to fulfil its function adequately.

Recent developments in immunology, psychology and the interdisciplinary field of psycho(neuro)immunology (PI) question these views. A model is defined as an explanation for phenomena that is revised or abandoned when it fails to account adequately for all the data. A dogma on the other hand requires that discrepant data be forced to fit the model or be excluded. Clearly, as scientists, we would acknowledge that our capacity to understand the immune system is benefited by adopting the former of the two approaches. But more than being prepared to work with new models, we should question the existing 'models' for elements of ingrained dogmatism.

THE NEURO-IMMUNE NETWORK AND PARACRINOLOGY

Such a reductionist model/dogma has, however, resulted in the research techniques that have elucidated the understanding we now have of the complexity of the immune system and its connections. The paracrine system was first described in 1938 by Friedrich Feytrer, a German pathologist, to explain his observation that some hormones are carried from one cell directly to a neighbouring cell (parallel cell) — hence the name paracrine system. The ongoing discovery of endocrine cells throughout the body and the brain provides us with a radical new model for understanding the possible connections between the previously partitioned 'systems'.

In the immune system alone, the communication and influence of cytokines (hormone-like mediators), antibodies and other molecules secreted by the various cells can, to some extent, be mapped with molecular biological techniques. The dynamic equilibrium observable within these self-regulating pathways can be disturbed by the introduction of foreign material, leading to the production of specific proteins (antibodies) to recognise and mark for destruction this introduced material, thus re-establishing a new balance. But in the complexity that becomes apparent in the interconnections of the 13-odd cytokines, these isolated effects are like the workings of a simple abacus in relation to a personal computer. This is made more so by the secretion of hormones previously thought only to be released by the pituitary, i.e. ACTH[3]. Even more so, as not only were they being secreted by immune cells but also by most other tissues in the body. Although the reductionist approach has led us to the ballgame of the body, it has no model to understand the rules by which it plays.

THE SYMPHONY OF EMOTIONS

The brain had always been thought of rather as an electrical computer system with commands going out to the body through the nerves, and also via some hormonal channels. Neurosurgeon Richard Bergland, in his book *The Fabric of Mind*[4], follows the history of this 'model' and tears it apart. We now know that the brain sends not only hormonal messages down nerves, but that it also receives information back from these same organs (just like the example of the testicle). He describes the mind/body interface as a symphony with a multitude of hormonal 'notes' being played to create the sensations of joy, hunger, anger, fatigue, etc. We know this because an analysis of teardrops confirms that the body has one chemistry for joy and another for sadness. The hormonal 'notes' include elements of the cytokine system, with larger notes being precursors for smaller notes with perhaps a totally different action. It may be that we will no longer be able to separate any of the various 'systems', but rather be forced to adopt an holistic model of function because we cannot understand the complexity of the interconnections in the dynamic state!

The problem is how or why do we all play our 'instruments' so differently when we would seem to have certain similar expectations. The answer is again based on models — models of human development based on inheritance and environment. We could argue, as have many before us, that one or the other plays the major role in moulding us as individuals. Whichever one plays the main role — and that may vary — forms us largely as individuals in our activities in life and our responses to life situations. Not too surprisingly, however, there are psychological categories that we *all* more or less fall into. One of the clearest ways to categorise a person is their response to stress.

STRESS AND IMMUNITY

'Stress' means all kinds of things, but essentially it is created by a situation in which we feel uncomfortable. A classic study done on medical students in the early 1980s focussed on exams as a psychological stressor[5]. More importantly, the study documented how stressed the students felt at this time. The results showed a clear correlation between the perceived stress and an increased incidence of illness and depressed immune states. The critical parameter here is the *perception* of stress as a marker of the physical response. All students are exposed to exams, but some have responses which don't affect their immunity while others are profoundly affected.

In a review of Chronic Fatigue Syndrome (CFS)[6], relapses were investigated as being precipitated by undue physical or mental stress. Dr Levy et al[7] published a paper documenting very clearly the correlation of stress factors and sustained depression of Natural Killer (NK) cells. These cells are one of the best indicators of the immune function's response to stress[5], and Dr Caligiuri et al were able to show the relationship between depression of the immune system and CFS[8]. A recent paper has summarised the effects of stress on the immune system[9]. How does stress create these effects?

Stress can be acute; the reactions to being badly frightened or to frequent driving in heavy traffic or to a work mate who constantly criticises include a racing heart, muscle tension, a dry mouth and a sense of panic. The reaction to acute stress would seem to have its origin in prehistory, with a need to be able to respond to life threatening situations by flight or fight. The adrenalin and cortisone released by the adrenal gland prepare the body for action, enabling it to perform amazing feats of survival. The feats are sometimes still seen today, for example, the lifting of a car by a normally built person after an accident. But the result of the release of these hormones in the twentieth century can have undesirable effects on immune function. Adrenalin, the major stress reactive hormone, allows fast adaptation to danger, overriding the body's usual regulatory mechanisms, but also releases a whole cascade of other hormones. There is good evidence to show that it changes the balance of lymphocytes released into the blood which, although poorly understood, may have short-term inhibiting effects.

In the longer term, release of corticosteroids inhibits the function of macrophages and lymphocytes and can affect the ability of lymphocytes to divide. These effects make corticosteroids powerful agents in allergic, arthritic and other immune dysfunctional states, in which the immune system is not functioning properly. But this immuno-suppression can lead to other problems. The basic response to chronic stress was originally described by Dr Hans Selye in the 1930s. Constant exposure to stress can cause hypertrophy or enlargement of the adrenal glands and atrophy or withering of lymphoid tissues.

Although we perhaps cannot say with certainty that these are the mechanisms, it helps us to understand why some individuals who don't 'cope' may become ill more often and illustrates how our thinking and feeling affect our health.

CONDITIONING THE IMMUNE SYSTEM

Research is showing that the immune system can be behaviourally conditioned. Multiple animal reports highlight the way in which the immune system can be manipulated[10-11]. In 1975 Robert Ader and his colleagues accidentally discovered that rats previously injected with cyclophosphamide and simultaneously fed saccharin-sweetened water became immunologically depressed when given saccharin alone. These findings have been repeated across the range of immunologic mediators, and these conditioned responses have been shown to affect the health and even survival of the experimental animals.

Successful conditioning of the *human* immune response (biofeedback and other techniques) has been less prolific, but significant nevertheless[12]. The results are important because they illustrate the possibility of regaining competent immune system function in diseases that we are now able to distinguish as immunologically affected if not mediated. It places also in context the findings about CFS, which show that our population is one in which immune potential is reduced. The cause of this may be the multitudinous factors mentioned in other sections of this book, but it may in fact be a result of CFS patients' experience of chronic ill health.

FATIGUE — PHYSICAL OR (NEUROGENIC) MENTAL

Chronic Fatigue Syndrome creates dilemmas for those researching it because it won't fit into a normal syndromic pattern. The criteria drawn up for diagnosing CFS are strict and, in one study at the University of Connecticut, of 135 patients complaining of chronic fatigue, only six qualified as having the syndrome. Although most of the studies on CFS describe a significant proportion of persons having an acute phase typical of a viral illness, there are a majority of patients who do not display such a clear physical basis. An acute phase followed by being unwell is understandable medically, for we can propose a residual viral problem that will recover over time if supportive therapy is provided. The other side of the coin is that:

- Most CFS patients show signs of depression
- The tendency to depression was not present any more than in the normal population before they became unwell
- There are clear indicators that symptomatology can be related to stress events
- Mental symptoms of anxiety, fastidiousness, poor self image, inflexibility, difficulty concentrating, dizziness, etc. exist.

Are these symptoms of a physical illness? Can we understand how such a plethora of symptoms can be boxed into CFS, a *syndrome*? A. R. Lloyd and his co-workers[13-14] have been working on this issue for some years now, trying to determine how psychological and immunological factors are related in CFS. Their hypothesis has been that CFS patients suffer from depression as a response to their life situation (so-called reactive or neurotic depression), with undue emphasis on somatic symptoms, particularly fatigue. The results of a trial comparing CFS patients with so-called people suffering from endogenous depression, in terms of their physical symptoms and their immunological parameters showed the two groups to be similar. Their most recent work has demonstrated a lack of muscle weakness in those with CFS fatigue. Dr Lloyd's team has contributed greatly to the medical acceptance of CFS, and their recent conclusion has been that CFS has a neurogenic basis. This takes us directly into the realms of viruses, chemicals, and metabolic disorders, etc., which we know from an accepted medical point of view affect the brain.

The biggest problem in doctors researching CFS is that they are looking for a single cause. This is a medical education problem, as we are taught in medical school that common things occur commonly, and hence we look for a single cause for a problem. What if the causes of CFS are as diverse as Dr Vayda's book suggests, and we are living in a polluted environment with which not all of us are metabolically adapted to cope? What if doctors and patients we have been slowly immunologically suppressed through the use of medicines we thought were beneficial? How can we understand the multiple causes if we don't stay open to all possibilities and work towards therapies that may not at this stage have mechanisms of action, but are at least helpful, if not curative?

A RESEARCH PROBLEM?

A mathematician called A. D. Allen, in a paper titled 'Left-right spatial agnosia and other mental defects that characterise clinical researchers'[15], clarifies the issue of the questions asked by researchers (logical significance) and the adequacy of the data in answering them (statistical significance). He claims that clinical researchers routinely make incorrect determinations as to their study's logical significance because of a spatial (left–right) agnosia. He goes on ...

> ... clinicians who have a useful insight or opinion to share should be able to publish it without having to conduct a study and without prejudice for not having conducted a study. Collecting data is not in itself science. The purpose of science is to find invariant phenomena hidden in diverse anecdotes that can be synthesized into a mathematical model (scientific theory) that helps us to understand, predict, and ultimately exercise some control over natural phenomena.

ANOTHER MODEL FOR POOR RESPONDERS

After we have carried out all the diagnostic and therapeutic measures outlined in this book, there will still probably be a group of non-responders who are difficult to understand even from a complimentary medical model. A non-mechanistic view of the condition includes the possibility of a physical trigger that lets the body know what it feels like to be unwell. This can go on for as long or as short a time as it takes a 'normal' person to recover. Some people, though, will be in a state or a life situation where stressors such as finance, exams, etc., may be affecting their immune systems; or they may be the type of person described earlier, who is unable to 'cope' with life situations, and is consequently set up for a protracted illness.

This occurs either through the persistence of immune compromising stressors or because the person starts to become focussed on their illness. This is described in psychological terms as becoming somatocentric, through a process called lateral inhibition. This occurs when anything that we're not paying attention to gets shut out and normally serves a protective function by allowing us to concentrate on certain things without being disturbed. It explains why, for example, we may not notice shoes on our feet until a nail comes through, then the shoes become central to our thinking until we can get them off, and the nail with them. By shutting off what we're not paying attention to, this process allows the focus to fill our conscious horizon to the exclusion of all else. In the words of Dean Black: 'Their physical problems get enlarged by worry and they get immobilised by exhausting despair.'

This can cause a vicious circle of being physically unwell at first, then, with time, a concentration on the physical and disabling mental symptoms increases, and life starts to revolve around the progress of how they feel. This robs them of friends, of interests, of stimulus to maintain basic health practices, and of the strength of purpose to stabilise their health, let alone to get well. Quite often rest can work wonders, if they can get any, but they usually find that if they try to go back to old activities, the old symptoms all come back.

CHRONICALLY UNWELL — NO NEW SYNDROME, BUT PERHAPS OLD CURES

CFS is not a new condition. As early as 1869 a psychiatrist, George Beard, coined neurasthenia as a term to describe chronic fatigue. Soon after, a neurologist 'developed' a rest cure, which involved a healthful diet, massage, complete rest and removal from the stresses of daily life, including family. As in more recent times, the diagnosis of a problem with so many symptoms in such non-perjorative terms became quite popular. Although the treatment was relatively successful, the problem of a specific diagnostic criteria still existed. As medicine became a science, it regarded the syndrome as a constitutional illness and lost interest. Such treatments are being utilised increasingly in this country, while they have long been a cultural feature in others. The yearly retreat to spas and sanatoriums is accepted practice in Europe, where clean air, rest, good food, physical therapies and a removal from mundane activities provide rejuvenation for tired workers.

Most often there is no time or money for such activities in our culture. The fact that states of mind can influence our susceptibility to disease, as well as our ability to get well again, creates a vital challenge for the medical profession. We should become better able to encourage attitudes that maximise homeostatic mechanisms.

CENTRES OF HEALING

If, as some people think, the major determinant in the pathogenesis of CFS is the patient's immune response, we are faced with the dilemma of treatment modalities for such a condition, at least from an orthodox medical perspective. On the other hand, if we treat fatigue as a sign of a problem and go searching for a cause, as we are trained to do, we can unearth many well documented and successful approaches. Some of these are becoming more acceptable[16], some are less mainstream. Even with the broadest physical and psychological modalities there are some failures. The most successful approach is a combination of all possible therapies, guided by someone experienced in the application of the various modalities, in combination with appropriate timing and combination.

This requires a centre with facilities for consultation, diagnosis and therapies. The program should combine the physical features with an appropriate re-conditioning of dietary, activity, social and personal habits. Meditation produces bodily changes that increase homeostatic rather than dysregulatory functions. Unfortunately, most people with CFS find it difficult to launch into anything regular. To start with weekly massage can be a gentle way of encouraging regularity and generating the relaxation response. Once there is an initial clearance of some of the most troubling symptoms, the building of a regular group activity has powerful long-term actions. The sense of security developed in regular meetings and working at learning to meditate, in encouraging one another to cope with the day-to-day restrictions of sensitivities and unpredictable illness, builds support structures not present in most suburban subcultures. Experienced facilitators constantly encourage activity outside personal boundaries so as to expand the constricted horizons closing in on those with moderate to severe illnesses.

The use of other more specific therapies, such as music, art and movement, works best in the hands of trained therapists, though their use is rare and requires more effort than the benefit gained. The results of such programs have been well documented[17], and present a great challenge for therapists and doctors to work together to provide a nurturing, mutually challenging environment.

HOW TO BE YOUR OWN BEST DOCTOR

This may seem to be a formidable task. How can you ever know enough to take that responsibility? Experience tells those of us that work in this area that patients who are keen to learn why they are unwell and who will unstintingly apply the principles that will help them at home, get the best results. The easier parts can be food restrictions and sleeping on a futon. It's the discipline of ordering your life and making time for self-healing activities that are the most difficult. Ultimately if you don't become your own best doctor, you will go on seeing endless other 'doctors'. Maybe you will find some relief in seeing them, but if you take the responsibility to learn and apply what you learn, you will get well. All the best.

References

1. Eysenck, H. J., 'Personality, Stress and Cancer: Prediction and prophylaxis', *B J Med Psy,* 1988: 61, 57–65
2. Booth, R., 'The Psychoneuroimmune network: expanding our understanding of immunity and disease', *New Zealand Journal of Medicine,* 1990 (to be confirmed)
3. Smith, E. M., Blalock, J. E., 'Human leucocyte production of ACTH and endorphin-like substances: association with leucocyte interferon, *Proc Nat Acad Sci USA,* 1981, 78: 7530–4
4. Bergland, R., *The Fabric of Mind,* Penguin, 1988
5. Kiecolt-Glaser, J., et al, 'Modulatio of cellular immunity in Medical Students', *Journal of Behavioural Medicine,* 1986, 9: 5–21
6. Archer, M. I., 'The post-viral syndrome: a review', *J RCGP,* 1987, 37: 212–214
7. Levy, S., et al, 'Correlation of stress factors with sustained depression of the Natural Killer activity and predicted prognosis in patients with breast cancer', *Journal of Clinical Oncology,* 1987, 5: 348–353

8 Caligiuri, M., et al, 'Phenotypic and functional deficiency of natural killer cells in patients with chronic fatigue syndrome', *Journal of Immunology,* 1987, 139: 3306–13
9 Khansari, R., et al, 'Effects of stress on the immune system', *Immunology Today,* 1990, 11: 5: 170–5
10 Ader, R., and Cohen, N., 'Behaviourally-conditioned immunosuppression', *Psychosom Med,* 1975, 37: 333–40
11 Kuscnecov, A. W., et al, 'Behaviourally conditioned suppression of the immune response by antilymphocyte serum', *Journal of Immunology,* 1983, 130: 2117–20
12 Smith, G. R. and McDaniel, S. M., 'Psychologically mediated effect on the delayed hypersensitivity reaction to tuberculin in humans', *Psychosom Med,* 1983, 45: 65–9
13 Lloyd, A. R., et al, 'Immunologic abnormalities in the chronic fatigue syndrome', *Medical Journal of Australia,* 1989, 151: 122–124
14 Lloyd, A., et al., Letter, *Medical Journal of Australia,* 1990, 152: 51
15 Allen, A. D., 'Left–right agnosia, and other mental defects that characterise clinical researchers', *Med Hypoth,* 1990, 31: 115–120
16 Siemensma, N. P., *Food Allergy and Intolerance,* Self-published
17 Earle, R., *Your Vitality Quotient: A program to build youth,* Warner Books, New York

How to Interpret Viral CFS Readings

During an acute attack of glandular fever the reading is likely to be:
- Anti-viral capsid antibodies (VCAs) will usually be positive, with their number usually high. The VCAs will usually remain positive for a long time, even after healing has occurred.
- Anti-Epstein-Barr Nuclear Antibodies (EBNAs) are usually negative at this stage but are likely to turn positive several months after the attack.
- Anti-Early-Antigens (EAs) can remain negative but often become positive within ten days or so.
- In such cases the IgM is also positive.

During a re-activation of the glandular fever virus some time later
Some time AFTER THE ORIGINAL ATTACK, if one has not been able to beat the virus into total withdrawal into the B cells and into a harmless state, the virus can be RE-ACTIVATED. As we have seen throughout this book, this can happen at any time as a result of many factors.

When this happens, and during the acute phase of such re-activation, the blood profile will change to:

- VCA: Positive — sometimes with high titres.
- EBNA: Positive or negative if it is the first such viral attack or if the assault was poorly handled by the immune system.
- EAs: Usually, but not always, positive.
- IgMs: Usually negative.

During chronic re-activation
If the virus has managed to conquer your defences and has established a chronic infection, the immune system may begin to show signs of disarray. The EBV profile may change as follows:

- VCA: Positive — usually with high titre counts (640 or more).
- EBNA: Can be positive but often remains negative if one is very ill.
- EAs: Positive but they can be alternating from positive to negative and back to positive for periods of time if the patient has relapses.

To the best of my knowledge this particular viral pathology is only available through Macquarie Pathology Services.

Some Useful Addresses

The Complementary and Environmental Medicine Centre
41 Boundary Street, Rushcutters Bay, NSW 2011
(02) 380 5233 and (02) 380 5474

The Environmental Medicine Centre, Manly Waters Private Hospital (Special Environment Allergy Centre)
17 Cove Avenue, Manly, NSW 2095
(02) 977 5577

Evandale Medical Chambers
45 Bundall Road, Surfers Paradise, Queensland 4217
(075) 38 2288

Macquarie Pathology (Head office in New South Wales)
35 Moore Street, Leichhardt, NSW 2040
(02) 692 7000

Macquarie Pathology Services has many branch offices throughout the Sydney metropolitan area and in New South Wales and parts of Queensland

Australian Research Laboratories
5 Levinson Street, North Melbourne, Victoria 3051
(03) 328 3586

Allersearch Asthma and Allergy Aids
8 Marco Avenue, Revesby, NSW 2212
(02) 771 6944

28 Martha Street, Granville, NSW 2142
(02) 637 8122

For controlling and eradicating dust mites and moulds

Envirotest
12 Don Young Street, Mount Gravatt Research Park, Nathan, Queensland 4111
(07) 343 6066

This group is currently working on simple methods to measure and detect dangerous levels of indoor pollution, as well as special equipment to purify the air xenobiotics, which should be available by the end of 1991

Interlight Australia
5 Hunter Street, Parramatta, NSW 2150
(02) 689 1542

Special electrostatic airfilters are available from Fred Vella (02) 823 7919

Glossary

Aceteldehyde An intermediate product of the breakdown of several chemicals and brain hormones. Also believed to be manufactured by *Candida albicans*. Highly toxic unless further metabolised and excreted

Adaptation The process by which the body learns to tolerate things and events that are potentially harmful to it. It is a stressful process for the body and therefore uses up energy and nutrients

Adaptogenic A word coined by Russian scientists to denote various 'tonics' that help the body adapt to various stresses.

Adrenalin Also known as epinephrine, it is the main stress response hormone. Sometimes called the 'fight or flight' hormone

Adrenal gland A gland involved in the hormonal responses to such factors as stress. Made up of a soft centre and an outer shell, each of these parts releases their own specific secretion

Alcohol dehydrogenase The principal enzyme that breaks down alcohol to its metabolite, aldehyde. It is an important enzyme in the first phase of detoxification and one that is believed to be present in lesser amounts in women. Because it is also part of the process by which the liver degrades chemicals, it may be responsible for the more noticeable mood-changing effects of chemical toxicity in women

Aldehyde A general category of intermediate products of the breakdown metabolism of many chemicals which are toxic if a bottleneck occurs at this point

Aldehyde dehydrogenase An enzyme that metabolises to 'safe' acids before excretion

Allergen Any substance which might cause an allergic reaction or intolerance

Allergy A hypersensitive reaction to things such as foods, chemicals, pollens, etc., which in other people cause no reaction

Amino acids The basic constituents of proteins

Antibiotics Chemicals which can inhibit the growth or destroy micro-organisms such as bacteria.

Antibody Part of the immune system formed to counteract viruses, bacteria and other micro-organisms that may cause illness

Antigens Substances which cause the production of antibodies

Autoimmunity The state in which a person becomes sensitised (perhaps 'allergic') to substances created in their own body.

Autoimmune disease A disease caused by an excess of autoimmunity

Basophils Part of the body's response to inflammation. They stain easily for identification

B cells Lymphocytes that produce antibodies, including immunoglobulins such as IgA and IgM, in response to a specific antigen

Biochemical individuality The understanding that every person's biology and biochemistry is different and will respond to different things in purely individual ways

Candida albicans A pathogenic yeast fungus which is usually harmless but can become dangerous to health if it is allowed to overgrow.

Carbon tetrachloride A component of solvents which is a powerful toxin, especially to the liver

Carcinogen An agent that may cause cancer

Carcinogenicity The potential of any particular substance to cause cancer

Catalise To help a process (biochemical) without undergoing destruction

Chelation therapy Intravenous infusion of substances which attach themselves to minerals and remove them from the blood

Chemical hypersensitivity Heightened sensitivity to one or several chemicals, frequently those that are common to our environment even in relatively small quantities

Conjugation The coupling of a chemical protein so it can be removed from the body. It is one of the detox systems

Cortisone A hormone produced by the adrenal cortex which is used in the treatment of many diseases, such as arthritis

Cross-linking The formation of abnormal chemical bonds that accelerate ageing. They can be caused by free radicals, chemicals, high blood sugar levels and a high consumption of sucrose or fructose (fruit sugar), especially on an empty stomach

Cytochrome P-450 The crucial enzyme that starts off the first phase of detoxification

Cytotoxic Anything which is toxic and usually lethal to a cell

DNA Deoxyribonucleic acid. The large molecules found in the nucleus of every cell that are responsible for containing and passing on all genetic characteristics of a lifeform

Dysbiosis An imbalance in the number and types of gut flora microorganisms, which cause various digestive processes to malfunction

Elimination diet Any form of diet that eliminates one or any substance for the nutritional consumption of an individual. Usually used in diagnosing and treating allergies or other illnesses that can be influenced by dietary intake

Endocrine gland Glands that secrete substances within the body

Endocrine system The system within the body that is made up of the organs and the related endocrine glands that act upon them

Endogenous pyrogen A fever inducing substance from within the body

Endoplasmic reticulum A set of membranes in the cell where detoxification occurs

End pointing A step in allergy-testing procedures at which the weal created by the skin reaction to the allergen being tested stops growing. Used to determine the strength of the allergy vaccine to be prepared

Enzyme Any protein that causes a chemical reaction that forms a necessary part in the proper functioning of cells

Environmental medicine A relatively new branch of medicine which concerns itself with the effects of the environment on human health

Ester The compound formed by removing water from the combination of acid and alcohol

Formic acid A metabolite of formaldehyde whose levels can be used to indicate if formaldehyde is being cleared adequately by the body

Gammaglobulin A blood protein

Glucocorticoids Hormones produced by the adrenal cortex in response to stress

Glutathione An essential part of the mechanism that conjugates chemicals so that the body can detox

Glutathion peroxidase A selenium-dependent enzyme that helps protect cell membranes from deterioration via oxidation of lipids (including polyunsaturated oils). As it neutralises peroxides it triggers glutathion to conjugate with and carry away the remaining leftovers of xenobiotics

Granulocytes Blood cells containing small particles

Histamine A substance released in the body as a response to some allergic reactions

Hypoglycemia Decreased sugar levels in the blood

GLOSSARY

Hypothalamus A small portion of the brain that correlates much of the information from outside and inside the body and sends signals to coordinate the activities of the nervous system and hormonal responses to these signals

Immune system The system in the body dedicated to protecting or defending the body from disease

Immunodeficiency A deficienct immune system

Immunoglobulin A group of molecules made from proteins that are part of the immune system's defence forces. Different immunoglobulins respond to different threats

Inert ingredients An advertising gimmick to make buyers believe the substance is harmless. In fact they often are the carriers of hydrocarbon solvents or pesticides. At times they can be more toxic than the actual pesticides

Intolerance A reaction that occurs but is not identifiable as an allergy by common immunological reactions

Intradermal Inside the skin

IVC Intravenous vitamin C Intravenous infusions in the form of drips, of vitamin C

Kinesiology The study of the mechanics of body movement

Kuppfer cells A group of liver cells which are part of that organ's antiviral activity. Part of the reticulo endothelial system (RES), they are known as macrophages elsewhere in the body

Lipids A general name for fats and oils

Lipid peroxidation Free radical attacks on cell membranes, such as occur in the lungs when you breath pollution, which can damage the cells and lead to chain destruction if not enough antioxidants are present

Lipid peroxides Free radicals that cause cell damage

Lymphadenopathy Swelling of the lymph nodes

Lymphoma Cancer of the immune system

Melanoma A malignant tumour derived from pigment containing cells

Metabolism The process by which substances such as nutrients are broken down and rebuilt in different forms composed of catabolism (breaking down) and anabolism (rebuilding)

Methacrylate A chemical that outgasses from plastic, adhesives and some material used in dentistry

Methemoglobimia A type of blood disorder that can be inherited but usually follows poisoning of the blood by some substances

Methylene chloride or dichloromethand A solvent used in paints, strippers, aerosol propellants and other products which can be metabolised by the body to carbon monoxide

Metabolite A substance acted upon or produced by metabolism

Mitochondria Membrane-encased cylindrical structures inside cells where energy is produced

Mutagens Substances that may cause genetic changes that can lead to cancer

Myocardial Of the heart muscles

Mycotoxins Fungi, moulds and the toxins that they can produce

Neuroendocrinal transducer Organ that translates inputs/signals (such as light, temperature, etc.) into nervous impulses, that in turn cause endocrinal glands to secrete hormones

Neuropathy Disease of the nervous tissue

Neuropsychiatry Dealing with diseases of the mind and nervous system

Neurotransmitter A chemical that carries, facilitates or inhibits messages from one brain cell to another

CHRONIC FATIGUE

Organophosphorous compounds   A common class of pesticides that are toxic to parts of the nervous system

Oxidation   The 'burning' process that is part of metabolism involved in the production of energy

Oxygen therapies   Treatment involving the use of oxygen compounds such as hydrogen peroxide and ozone

Paresthesia   A tingling or numbness of extremities

Pancreas   An endocrine gland which secretes a digestive fluid into the intestine and which also produces insulin

Parathyroid   Small glands situated near the thyroid gland which secrete a substance that controls the level of calcium in the blood

Patch test   An allergy test which tests reactions to potential allergens on the skin

Pathogenic   Disease producing

pH level   The measure of acidity or alkalinity in the body: the normal balance is 7

Phytates   Substances in some undercooked or raw vegetables and grains that can inhibit mineral absorption from food

Pineal gland   A gland of the endocrine system located in the brain that interacts between inputs from the environment and the secretions of many hormones

Pituitary gland   A gland of the endocrine system located at the base of the brain that controls most, if not all, the endocrine secretions

Plasma   The liquid portion of the blood

Probiotics   The antithesis of antibiotics — substances that are life encouraging

Pulse test   Measurement of the change in pulse rate caused by allergic reaction

Redox ability/index   A measure of the capacity to balance or neutralise the body chemistry so as to minimise free radical formation

Solvents   A substance that has the power to dissolve another

Styrene   A potentially carcinogenic material used to make such items as plastic cups. Excreted in the urine as mandelic acid. Increased blood levels of this chemical have been found in people after they drink hot beverages from styrene cups

Sublingual   Situated or placed under the tongue

Systemic candidiasis   A potentially serious condition in which candida organisms have invaded many parts of the human system simultaneously

Tachycardia   An abnormally fast heart beat, as distinct from palpitations, which often include irregular heartbeats

Thymus gland   A gland located in the chest that trains the various soldiers of the immune army during the early years of life

Thyroid   A neck gland

Toluene and xylene   Relatives of benzene, they are solvents that outgass from products like paints. Measured in the urine as hippuric acid

Topical   Applied to a particular location on the skin

Trichloroethylene (TCE) and tetrachloroethylene   Ubiquitous solvents used in many industrial processes, including dry-cleaning**Vinyl chloride**   Outgassings from plastics. Sometimes responsible for TBC (toxic brain syndrome) symptoms

Volatile compounds   Substances that get into the air which can be inhaled via the lungs, thus allowing entry to the bloodstream and brain

Xenobiotics   A foreign chemical

Xenobiotic overload   An excess amount of xenobiotics

Bibliography

Appelboom, T., and Flowers, F., 'Ketonconazole in the treatment of chronic mucocoutaneous candidiasis secondary to autoimmune polyendocrinopathy-candidiasis syndrome', *Cutis*, 1982, 30:71-2

Arulanantham, K., Dwyer, J. M., and Genl, M., 'Evidence for defective immunoregulation in the syndrome of familial candidiasis endocrinopathy', *New England Journal of Medicine*, 1978, 300 (4) 164-8

Bahn, A. K., et al., 'Hypothyroidism in workers exposed to polybromated biphenyls', *New England Journal of Medicine*, 1980, 320:31

Beisel, William R., et al., 'Single-nutrient effects on immunologic functions', *Journal of the American Medical Association*, 245:1, p. 53, 1981

Bharati, C. Purohit, et al., 'The formation of germatures by *Candida albicans* when grown with *Staphilococcus pyogenes*, *Escherichia coli*, *Klebsiella pneumoniae*, *Lactobacillus acidophilus* and *Proteus vulgaris*', *Mycopathologie*, Vol. 63:3, 1977

Boyne, R. and Arthur, J.R., 'The response of selenium deficient mice to *Candida albicans* infection', Rowlett Research Institute, Scotland, Communication, 1989

Brostoff, Dr J. and Challacombe, Dr S. J., *Food Allergies*, Bailliere Tindall, London, 1987

Crook, Dr William, *The Yeast Connection*, Professional Books, Jackson, Tennessee 1983

Dempsey, A., DeSwiet, M. and Dewhurst, J., 'Premature ovarian failure associated with candida endocrinopathy syndrome', *British Journal of Obstetrics and Gynaecology*, 1981

Dokn, J., Varma, S. and South M.A., 'Chronic mucocutaneous candidiasis endocrinopathies', *Cutis*, 27:592, 1981

Englard, Sasha and Seifter, Sam, 'The biochemical functions of ascorbic acid', *Annual Review of Nutrition*, 6:365-406, 1986

Gerard, John W., *Food Allergy*, Charles C. Thomas, Illinois, 1980

Halpern, M. J. and Durlock, M. J. (eds), *Magnesium Deficiency*, S. Karger, Switzerland, 1985

Hathcock, J. N. (ed.), *Nutritional Toxicology* (Vol. 2), Academic Press, Florida, 1987

Huwyler, Toni, et al., 'Effect of ascorbic acid on human natural killer cells', *Immunology Letter*, 10:173-76, 1985

Jakoby, William B., *Enzymatic Basis of Detoxification* (Vols 1 and 2), Academic Press, New York, 1980

Jakoby, W. B., Bent, J. and Caldwell, J., *Metabolic Basis of Detoxification*, Academic Press, New York, 1982

Kaffe, S., Petigrew, C. S., et al., 'Variable cell-mediated immune defects in a family with candida endocrinopathy syndrome', *Clinical Experiments Immunology*, 20:397-408, 1975

Kennedy, Michael and Volz, Paula A., 'Exology of *Candida albicans* gut colonization: Inhibition of candida adhesion, colonization and dissemination from the gastrointestinal tract by bacterial antagonism', *Journal of the American Society for Microbiology, Infection and Immunity*, 1985

Kenny, F. J. and Holliday, M., 'Hypothyroidism, moniliasis, Addison's and Hashimoto's diseases', *New England Journal of Medicine*, 27 (4):708-13, 1964

Kroker, George F. (ed), *Chronic candidiasis and Allergy. Food Allergy and Intolerance*, Bailliere Tindal, London, 1988

Kurttio, P., et al., 'Environmental and biological monitoring of exposure to ethylenebisdithiocarbamate fungicides and ethyenethiourea', *British Journal of Industrial Medicine*, 47:203-206, 1990

Levine, Steven, *Anti-oxidant Adaptation — Its Role in Free Radical Pathology*, Allergy Research Group, California, USA, 1985

Lewin, Roger, 'A new type of genetic disease', *New Scientist*, 30 June 1990

Mackarness, Dr R., *Not All in the Mind — The Hazards of Hidden Allergies*, Pan, London, 1976

Martin, E., *Hazards of Medication*, J. B. Lippincott, Toronto, London, 1978

Mathur, S., et al., 'Anti-ovarian and anti-lymphocyte antibodies in patients with chronic vaginal caindidiasis', *Journal of Reproductive Endocrinology*, 2:247, 1980

Miller, Thomas E. and North, Dereck K., 'Clinical infections, antibiotics and immunosuppression: a puzzling relationship', *Australian Journal of Medicine*, Vol. 71, 1981

Newbold, Dr H., *Revolutionary New Discoveries About Weight Loss*, Rawson, New York, 1977

Odds, F., Evans, et al., 'Prevalence of pathogenic yeasts and humoral antibodies to candida in diabetic patients', *Journal of Clinical Pathology*, 31:840-4, 1978

Okechukwu, Ekenna, et al., 'Factors affecting colonization and dissemination of *Candida albicans* from the gastrointestinal tract of mice', *American Society for Microbiology, Infection and Immunity*, July 1987, pp. 1558-63

Oldstone, Professor M., 'Viral Alteration of Cell Functions' *Scientific American*, August 1989

O'Shea, Dr James A., et al., 'The value of RAST tests in the diagnosis and treatment of multiple immune disorders, Twenty-second Scientific Session of the American Academy of Environmental Medicine, October 1988

Passwater, Richard, *Supernutrition for Healthy Hearts*, Dial Press, New York, 1977

Phaosawadst, Kamthorn, et al., 'Primary and secondary candida respohagitis in normal, healthy subject', Original Communication, June 1986

Piccoella, Enza, et al., 'Generation of suppressor cells in the response of human lymphocytes to a polysaccaride from *Candida albicans*', *Journal of Immunology*, 126:6, June 1981

Platt, Dr Stephen, 'Sickness linked to mould', Report on research at Royal Edinburgh Hospital, reported in *Sun Herald*, Sydney, 23 July 1989

Queen, Harold, *Chronic Mercury Toxicity*, Health Communication, Colorado, 1988

Rivas, Victor and Rogers, Thomas J., 'Studies on the cellular nature of *Candida albicans*-induced suppression', *Journal of Immunology*, 130:1, January 1983

Ryan, Mary, et al., 'Recurrent vaginal candidiasis: the importance of an intestinal reservoir', *Journal of the American Medical Association*, 238:17, 24 October 1977

Saltarelli, Professor C., *Candida albicans: The Pathogenic Fungus*, Hemisphere, New York, 1990

Schwartz, Dr G., *Food Power*, McGraw Hill, New York, 1979

Shakman, R., *Poison Proof Your Body*, Arlington, USA, 1980

Short, Dr Kate, *The A-Z of Chemicals in the Home*, Total Environment Centre, Sydney, 1989

Stoff, Dr Jesse A., *Chromic Fatigue Syndrome*, Harper and Row, New York, 1989

Trowbridge, Dr J.P., *The Yeast Syndrome*, Bantam, 1988

Vayda, William, *Are You Allergic to the Twentieth Century?*, Thomas Nelson, Melbourne, 1979

Vayda, William, 'Post Viral Syndrome and IVC', *Australian Wellbeing*, No. 22, 1987

Weiner, H. and Flynn, T. G., 'Enzymology and Molecular Biology of Carbonyl Metabolism, Aldehyde Dehydrogenase, Aldo-Reto Reductase, and Alcohol Dehydrogenase', *Journal of Biology*, Vol. 232, Alan R. Liss Inc., New York, 1987

Williams, Dr Roger, *You Are Unique*, Pitman, New York, 1971

Witkins, Steve S., et al., 'Inhibition of *Candida albicans*-induced lymphocyte proliferation by lyphocytes and sera from women with recurrent vaginitis', *American Journal of Obstetrics and Gynaecology*, 147:809, 1983

Yudkin, Dr J., *Sweet and Dangerous*, Bantam Books, New York, 1972

Zamm, A., *Your House May Endanger Your Health*, Simon and Schuster, New York, 1980

Zouali, Moncef, et al., 'Evaluation of auto-antibodies in chronic mucocutaneous candidiasis without enocrinopathy', *Mycopathologia*, 84:87, 1984

Index

Acquired immunity, 23
AIDS virus, 23, 30, 75, 77, 80, 147, 210, 211, 227
Allergies and CFS, 138-49
  allergic reaction, 138-9
  allergy, definition, 139-40
  allergy testing, 145
  changing face of allergy, 140-2
  dust mites, 146, 147, 149
  food cravings, 144-5
  food families, 142-4
  fungi, 146, 148-9
  glucose tolerance test, 145
  hypoglycaemia, 144
Allergy, 98, *see also* Allergies and CFS
  definition, 139
  pesticides, 126, 127
  weight problems, 183
Aluminium, 118
Alzheimer's disease, 43
Amino acids, 33, 102, 160, 174, 196
Antibiotics, 151, 160
Antioxidant metabolism, 63
Antioxidants, 31, 61, 63
Anxiety syndrome, 70
Arsenic, 123
Asthma, 71, 146-7, 148
Autoimmune diseases, 57, 138, 145, 171, 179
Autoimmune, Polyendocrinopathy, Immune Dysregulation, Candidiasis, Hypersensitivity Syndrome (APICHS), 59, 65, 87, 152, 169-71, 174
Bacteria, 17, 18, 20, 21
Biochemical individuality, 34-42
  diet, 38-40
  environmental medicine, 96
  enzymes, 37-8
  mutation, 37
  nutritional medicine, 40
  nutritionists, 41-2
  personalised reaction to food, 34-6
  pesticides, 126
  recommended daily allowances, 36
  sensitivities, 36-7
Body detoxification system, 101
  damage, 103
  detox pathway bottlenecks, 103
  phases, 102
  xenobiotics, 101, 103
Boron, 123

Cadmium, 123

Candida albicans, 21, 56, 58-60, 61, 64, 65, 76, 84, 85, 86, 89, 98, 107, 172, 175, 179, 180, 203, 222
  allergies, 138, 140, 148
  mercury, and, 120
Candida and CFS, 149-169
  allergies to candida, 155
  diagnosis, 157-8
  examination, 156
  symptoms of candida infection, 154-5
  tests
    candida antibodies 157
    CMI, 157
    culture, 157
    RAST, 156
    VEGA, 156
  treatment
    elimination diet, 158, 162-4
    general guidelines, 167
    making diets more interesting, 166
    MEVY diet, 166
    nutritional requirements, 160-2
    Nystatin powder, 158-9, 168
    vaginal/genital thrush, 168-9
Chemical CFS
  anti-pollutant guide, 135
  diet, 134-7
  basic rules, 109-11
  body detoxification system, 101-4
  checklist, 111
  chemical toxicity, 106-9
  environment, 91
    chemicals, 91-2, 93, 94
    diagnosis, 95
    Toxic Brain Syndrome, 95
    xenobiotics, 92
  environmental illness, 99, 100, 106
  environmental medicine, 96-9
    chemical overloading, 98-9
    environmental pollution, 96
    xenobiotics, 96
  home or workplace, 132
    common indoor pollutants, 132-3
    plant power, 134-5
    safe personal environment, 134
    sick building syndrome, 132
    UFFI exposure, 132
  neurotoxins, 112-26
  pesticides, 126-32
  tired or toxic, 100
    body detoxification system, 101
    detox pathway bottlenecks, 103, 105
    disappearance of symptoms, 104-6

Chemical Hypersensitivity Syndrome
  (CHS), 215
Chemical overloading, 65, 99-100, 106,
  153, 195
Chemical toxicity
  reduce exposure, 108
  suspecting, 107
  treatment, 108
Chemicals, 17, 21, 72, 84, 123
  depression, and, 178
  exposure, 141
  food addiction, 191
Chlorine, 123
Cholesterol, 56, 119
Chromic Candidiasis Sensitivity
  Syndrome, 155
Chronic Epstein Barr Virus Syndrome
  (CEBVS), 56, 57, 58, 65, 74, 153, 215
Chronic Fatigue Syndrome (CFS)
  chemical CFS, *see* Chemical CFS
  classification, 54
  depression, *see* Depression and CFS
  diagnosis, 63-72, *see also* Diagnosis,
    principles and methods; Diagnosing CFS
  emotionally unstable, 59
  environmental or viral, 72-3
  immunological abnormalities, 73
  modern medicine, and, 208-16
  onset of CFS, 63
  puzzle of CFS, 55-6
    candida, 58-60
    latent virus, 56
    viruses, 56-8
    xenobiotics, 60-3
  Special Environment Allergy Clinic
    (SEAC), 215
  suspecting you have CFS, 65-6
  symptoms, 54, 64-6, *see also*
    Symptoms of CFS
  treating, *see* Treating CFS
  typical symptomatology, 216, *see also*
    Typical symptomatology of CFS
  viral CFS, *see* Viral CFS
  viral or environmental, 72-3
Copper, 123

Dental mercury, 119, 120, 121
Depression and CFS, 70, 112, 172-81
  causes, 174
  chemicals, and, 178-80
  common symptoms, 172
  kinds, 173
  light, 176-8

  pineal gland, 176-7
  SADS, 176-8
  treatment, 174-5
  types, 172-3
Diagnosing CFS, 66-72, 85, 216, 219
  allergies and sensitivities, 71
  Candida antibodies test, 72
  gastrointestinal symptoms, 70
  lymph node swellings, 71
  muscular symptoms, 70
  neuropsychiatric symptoms, 70
  tests, 71
  tiredness, 72
Diagnosis, principle and methods, 219
  application and interpretation of tests
    Epstein Barr Virus, 225
    multitest CMI, 224
  proposed causes, 226
    allergy and intolerance, 228
    cellular damage, 227
    chemical hypersensitivity syndrome,
      228
    chemical toxicity, 228
    chronic opportunist infections, 227
    hormonal dysregulation, 228
    immunological disorder, 227
    nutritional deficiency, 228
    psychological stress, 228
  supportive findings, 220
    agents causing health problems, 221
    candidiasis, 222
    hormonal dysregulation, 223
    initial investigation, 220
Diet, 17-8, 33, 38-40, 129, 174
  anti-pollutant, 135
  chemical poisoning, and, 129
  elimination diet, 158, 162-4
  making interesting, 166
  MEVY diet, 164
  stress, and, 52
  treating, CFS, 196, 204
Dust mites, 71, 146, 147-9

Endocrine system, 46-9
Environment, 17, 91
  chemical sensitivity, 93-4
  chemicals, 91-2, 94
  diagnosis, 95
  environmental or viral CFS, 72-3
  Toxic Brain Syndrome, 95
  toxins, and, 115
Environmental Protection Association
  (USA), 132

INDEX

Epstein Barr virus, 32, 76-84, *see also*
  Chronic Epstein Barr Virus Syndrome
    (CEBVS)
  allergies, 141
  antibody studies, 225
  cancer, 83-4
  chemicals, 84
  glandular fever, 77, 79, 81
  herpes, 83
  history, 82
  lymphoma, 82-3
  measurement, 76, 78
  modern medicine, 214
  stress, 84
  treating CFS, 205
  viral screening, 85
Exercise, 31, 67

Fasting, 67
Foods for moods, 42-5
Formaldehyde, 98, 132, 135, 147
Fungi, 59, 60, 71, 110, 146, 148-9

Gamma Globulin (GG), 32
Glandular fever, 77, 79, 81
Gut flora, 31, 71

Human B-lymphotropic virus (HBLV), 81, 84
Human herpes 6 virus, 84
Human Immunodeficiency Virus (HIV), 210, 211
Hyperactivity, 143
Hypoglycemia, 59, 86, 144
Hypothalamus, 181, 182

Immune system, 191-34
  alteration of immune system, 25-7
  antigen presenting cells, 24
  antigens, 21
  antiviral measures, 26
    drugs, 26
  autoimmunity, 25
  basophils, 23
  candida, 59
  cell-mediated immunity, 20
  cells of the immune system, 63
  disrupting the immune system, 25
    drugs, 26
    stress, 26
    vaccination, 26
    viral infections, 25
    xenobiotics, 26
  excessive activity, 25
  exercise, 31-2
  fungi, 60
  granulocytes, 23, 24
  how the system works, 20, 23
  immunocompetence, 22
  Lactate Induced Anxiety Syndrome, 32
  lymphocytes, 21-2, 23-4
  macrophages, 20, 23, 30
  major histocompatibility complex, 24
  monocytes, 23
  neutrophils, 23
  non-specific immunity, 20
  oesinophils, 23
  protection of immunity, 27-31, 33
  stress, 26, 33
  temperature changes, 27
  toxic chemicals, 33
Immunocompetence, 22, 143
Intravenous Vitamin C therapy, 197-8

Lactate Induced Anxiety Syndrome, 32, 64, 70
Lead poisoning, 115
Liver, 66, 87-90
  treating CFS, 196
Lymphocytes, 21-2, 23-4, 62, 237
Lymphoma, 82

Manganese, 122, 123
Manic Depressive Psychosis, 173
Mercury, 118-21, 123
  dental, 119, 120, 121
  poisoning, 119, 125
  vegetarians, and, 119
Metabolism
  antioxidants, 63
  free radicals, 61-3
Methamyl poisoning, 131
Mucus, 30
Multitest CMI, 224

Natural immunity, 23
Neurotoxins, 112-126
  additives, effect, 123
  aluminium, 118
  avoiding effects, 124
  brain functions, 113
  chemicals, effect, 123
  depression, 112
  elimination, 125
  immune system, 112
  impairment of functions, 114

manganese, 122, 123
mercury, 118, 123
    candida, and, 120
    cholesterol, 119
    vegetarians, 119
nervous system, 112
nitrates, 117, 123
pollution, effect, 123
selenium, 121, 123, 125
toxins and the environment, 115
    trichloroethane, 122
    volatile fuels, 117
Neurotransmitters, 42, 43
Nickel, 123
Nitrates, 117, 123
Nutritional medicine, 40
Nutritionists, 41

Organophosphates, 128
Oxidation, 62
Oxygen therapies, 196

Pesticides, 126-132
Phthalates, 99
Pineal gland, 176-7
Plant power, 134-5
Pollution, 97, 123
    common indoor pollutants, 132
    effects, elimination, 124
Post partum depression, 173
Post Viral Syndrome, 56, 57, 58, 59, 65, 74, 153, 180
Profound Sensitivity Syndrome (PPS), 179
Psychodietetics, 45
Psychoneuroimmunologist, 55
Psychoneuroimmunology 232-44
Radio Allergo Absorbent Test (RAST), 72, 73, 86, 156

Seasonal Affective Disorders Syndrome (SADS), 173, 176-8
Selenium, 122, 124, 126
Stress, 18, 26, 33, 45-53, 73, 84, 183, 192
    depression, 174
    endocrine gland, 47
    hypothalamus, 47
    immunity, and, 236
    non-specific responses, 46
    oxidative, 63
    phases, 49-50
    pituitary gland, 47
Symptoms of CFS, 54, 64-6, 216

Tapanui Flu, 54
Therapeutic intervention, 229-31
Tin, 123
Titres — Viral footprints, 85-6
Total load, 18, 96
Toxic Brain Syndrome, 95
Toxicology, 115
Toxins, 115-24
    environment, and, 115
Treating CFS, 194-207
    basic principles, 200-4
    diets, 195-6
    intravenous vitamin C therapy, 197, 205
    oxygen therapies, 197, 205
    solutions not problems, 204-7
    supplements, 195
    therapeutic intervention, 229-31
    treatments, 199
        regimens, 204
Trichloroethane, 123
Trichloroethylene, 93, 135
Typical symptomatology of CFS, 216, 219
    intercurrent medical condition, 218
    218

Universal Reactivity Syndrome, 153
Urea Foam Formaldehyde Insulation (UFFI), 132

Viral CFS, 74-90
    diagnosis, 73, 85, 245
        titres, 85-6, 245
    Epstein Barr virus, 76-84
    liver, 87-90
    test results, 87, 245
    symptoms, 86
    viruses, 74-6
Virus, 17, 74
Volatile fuels, 117

Weight problems and CFS, 181-93
    allergy, 183
    hypothalamus, 181, 182
    obese child, 183
    regulation of food intake, 181
    stress, 183
    thermogenesis, 182
    type A eaters, 183-8
    type B obesity, 188-93

Xenobiotics, 26, 60-3, 90, 92, 96, 101, 103, 109-10, 123, 148, 170, 179